The First
100 DAYS

By Sheena Nicole

The First 100 Days. Copyright@2020 Sheena Nicole

www.getyouvisible.com

www.getyouvisible.com

ISBN: 978-1-989848-01-2

To my two beautiful sons. May you never read this.

The First 100 Days.

Here's an honest opinion of how it goes down.

Contents

Foreword.

This book, as the title suggests, speaks to the realness that occurs when a mother brings home her new baby. Sheena Nicole touches on the difficulties of childbirth, living with a new human, and everything messy in between. Her humour will keep readers engaged all while being able to relate to the general, bloody and disgusting truth about what women experience and what is not talked about when people on the outside think about the beauty of childbirth and babies. Being a new mother is hard and Sheena brings to light the not so perfect realities and downright chaos and insanity that is motherhood.

Sheena and I have been friends for many years. I too, am a mother. I can connect with her and relate to her struggles. Having been alongside her during her devastating miscarriages, I have felt both her pain as well as her bravery and determination. I can honestly say that she is one of the strongest women I know. Not only has she lived through the events that most women fear; she never gave up. She came through all the fog and bullshit to achieve her second living baby, and carry on with her life—scars and memories included. What was most incredible was how she carried those scars and living nightmares and put them into words to share with the world. Her vulnerability is what makes her beautiful.

The words in this book are true and relatable. How Sheena acknowledges what we struggle with, accomplish, fail at, and create as women is incredibly powerful. It is a long overdue and invaluable read that will allow mothers to feel worthy and connected.

Agnieszka D.
Registered Psychologist
Mom of two

Introduction.

The First 100 Days. It's the title that I ended up defaulting to for this book when I was reflecting on the time that follows the delivery of our babies. You know, the acute, torturous post-birth stint that mothers must endure before finally being able to feel like themselves again. I probably couldn't think of a better title. Actually, that might not be true. I had a lot of good ideas that I debated calling this sad soul of a novel, mostly with foul language and a darkened twist. But I did not want this book to portray negativity, because that is not what this book is about. The point of this book is to speak to the realness that occurs following childbirth and the raw reality that is mandatorily adopted by us, as mothers.

My intent was to uplift those reading this book, in such a way that we could find commonality between us. If there is any underlying theme that is true to this slightly offside novel, it is of empowering women to acknowledge their strength and resilience as we, together, survive these first 100 days.

As I find time to write this book, somewhere between shitty diapers and demanding household chores, my son is well past the 100-day mark and I still find myself ripping my hair out and chugging copious glasses of red wine in the closet. 100 days have passed since the birth of my son, isn't it supposed to be getting better now? I am referring to life in general, when we as women can regain our lives back; the freedom to put our babies to bed at 7:00 p.m. and not have to see their dirty little faces for another twelve hours. Don't get me wrong, we love our little ones, but it would be nice to have sex again with the lights on, not feeling guilty about the little mini-me staring over at us like a deer in the head lights.

When my little one was born and exhaustion had immediately taken over, a good friend of mine said to me: "The first week is the toughest! Hang in there, you've got this!" *Okay*, I thought, *seven days, that will fly by. I got this - I can do seven days.* But not long after that, I was informed: "You just gotta get through these first six weeks. The first six weeks are the hardest." *Okay*, I thought. *I can do that. Seven days ~ six weeks, potato potahto, right?* (Insert eye roll here.)

Six weeks isn't too bad considering how fast life flies in general, and even torn to shreds and ripped apart after what we call a *miracle*, I could envision the light at the end of that short six-week tunnel. But as the days passed and that six-week marker approached, nothing had seemed to substantially improve. Life still sucked, screaming baby still existed, sleepless nights still occurred, and one hormonal bitch of a mother was still present.

Someone else said to me: "You just gotta get over that eight-week hump, sister!" *Eight weeks now? Hmm, okay. So only two more weeks to go. I can do this! Let's think positive.* To which then I heard, oh yes, wait for it: "Just get to the three-month mark. It gets better after that. Those first three months are the worst." Then that clever optimistic piece of advice became six months, which extended to a year. You can probably see the pattern here and can probably guess what I was thinking: *when the hell does this end?* Someone, too, then joked that I will be able to sleep after eighteen years pass. *Thanks for the bloody joke, you moron, can I take my million-dollar rental of a breast pump and slap you with it?*

I quickly came to the realization that it probably never does *actually* end. It will always be one thing after another, and as the blessed chosen ones, we, as mothers, are going to have to be there for our children every day of their lives - for different reasons, of course. *Just get through these next eighteen years* seemed all too daunting to focus on, so I chose to stick with this initial phrase: that The First 100 Days are the most challenging, after which life will slowly and hopefully start to get a little easier, one day and one dirty diaper at a time.

Initially, I was tempted to title this book *6,570 days of Hell*, given that the little buggers will move out of the house on their eighteenth birthday. Better yet, *A Lifetime of Fucking Madness.* But, given the thought that if enough people read this book the world has a probable chance of never again re-populating, I thought that The First 100 Days would be the best place to start. Besides, The First 100 Days are the ugliest, most filthy of them all. And they truly do get better.

If you can get through these first 100 days, you will survive every single day after that.

Expert Opinion.

It is heartbreaking to see new moms in the clinic feeling ashamed that their postpartum experience does not feel as idyllic and blissful as they imagined it would. Labour and delivery are the biggest energy expenditures in a woman's life and are followed immediately by the huge transition into parenting. It can be a hard, scary time made much worse by our expectations that it should be delightful and perfect.

The First 100 Days is raw, real and honest. Sheena normalizes the REAL postpartum experience with detailed descriptions of the highs and lows women can expect when having a baby. Get ready for a wild ride, ladies. This book will make you gasp and cringe, laugh and cry but mostly it will validate you and your experience and help you know that you are not alone.

Dr. Jennifer D., R.Ac, TCMD, FABORM
Doctor of Traditional Chinese Medicine

Intention.

This book is intended for anyone who has kids, anyone who wants kids, for anyone who is pregnant, and for every sad soul who is somewhere between that birth and 100-day mark. Together, we can hash out the gruesome details and the *truth* about postpartum. None of that fairy-tale-la-da-da *bullshit* that people sugar-coat and feed to you, 'cause let's face it, ladies, whoever tells you that childbirth and postpartum experiences are fucking rainbows and flying cotton-candy eating fucking unicorns are flat out lying to you.

Together we will laugh, cry, agree, curse, feel sorry for ourselves, cry some more, slap our husbands, eat some ice cream (I prefer caramel with chocolate chips), and be the hormonal mammals that just birthed small miracles. We are women and we are emotional. Get over it. Accept it. Own it. It is perfectly okay to feel frustrated, overwhelmed, and even tearful during a commercial of *Keeping up with the Kardashians*. It is our body's fucked up reaction to the indescribable gift of childbirth that we just underwent.

Our emotions will have a mind of their own for a while. They will be loud and they will be dominant. They will make us feel defeated, crazy and not good enough, but they will not last forever. So, know that it's okay to cry at random points throughout the day. Understand that it's normal to feel overwhelmed with rage and guilt and upset all at the same time. Know that it's okay to not be able to understand and rationalize everything. Know that your emotions are real; that they are normal.

Try and be okay with letting it out, ladies. Cry because those fucking nipples hurt, and you have no idea what else to do with them. Scream into the pillow because you're mad at your partner for your significant vaginal distress (actually, even slap or give him the silent treatment for never again being able to live with that previously tight vagina). Release the anger from thinking about all that weight you've gained. And, if you don't have an explanation for the pitiful mess that you are currently displaying, then just sit with that. Let the emotions do their thing - they are going to anyway. Sit with it, be patient with it, and try to be kind to yourself for all of the changes that your body is undergoing and trying to regulate. And, for the good Lord's sake, *don't forget the ice cream.*

As awful as it seems, do not think for one second that we are bashing our young ones. We love our babies. Let's get that straight. We live for them. Every ounce of our existence goes into them and their wellbeing. They are our blood, our soul, and a true testament to our character. They truly do contribute to our happiness and stand for every single thing that we live for. But just because our children suddenly come into our lives, does not mean that the aftermath of birth and delivery is a pleasant one.

This book is not intended to be negative. It is meant to be real. Our children do not depict the hormonal tornado that comes with them. We love our children, but we do not have to like everything that comes along with that. It's okay to acknowledge that life is hard, that it is challenging, and that it is exhausting. Perhaps there is strength in voicing those challenges. Maybe by reading books similar to this one, women all over (and men too) can connect with the similar journeys of others. Maybe we can put the intimidating picture-perfect Betty fuckin' Crocker Instagram moms aside for a second - like, we get it Linda, you *make flawless cookies for your kid's birthday parties* - and come to the realization that we are more similar than different, that we all experience unpleasant emotions, and that we often feel alone more times than talked about.

We are all mothers, and we are more similar than different.

This book is intended to not only high five the fabulous and courageous women for completing the most incredible miracle of life, it is also here to let you know that you are not alone. *Together*, we will learn that everything we think, feel, and experience is normal. This shit happens. It's real. As beautiful as life is, it can be pretty dark and disgusting too, but we will get through these first 100 days, together. Trust me. We are women, and we are strong. We will kick postpartum's ass.

11

Even though the language is foul, and the visuals may be slightly disturbing, this book is coming from a good place - one of truthfulness, love, and gratitude. A place where we, as women, can be honest about the child birthing journey and what truthfully happens when we become parents to dirty little strangers.

Disclaimer: There is a lot of swearing in this book. If you are easily offended or highly opinionated, I would suggest you stop reading this book now. Put this book down, walk an aisle over, and go grab a copy of How to Bead Jewellery or Jungle Animals of the Dark or some shit, I don't care. Whatever.

But, if you are in for a good read about powerful women and the body's extraordinary capabilities, yours included, then set all judgement aside and allow yourself to indulge in a little potent humour. The words in this book are generalized, yet not exclusionary to any one person's experience with their own birthing journey. This has been my own personal experience of bearing children and I want to share it with those who might find any little bit of it helpful. It's simple. Kick back, read, enjoy. Take what you need – leave what you don't.

Oh, and by the way, as I write this book, I am somewhere in between sleep deprivation, regulating my hormones, re-introducing my period, and in somewhat of a drunken state. So, know that this book is not meant to be super structured in any way. It is not meant to even make complete sense at any given random time. It is as dishevelled as the lady writing it. I am not an author. I am not famous. I am not rich. This is me, as described a couple sentences ago, bearing my soul through words in what I have experienced along my birthing and parenting journeys. I am not asking to be judged. I frankly don't give a shit. I have judged myself enough along the way; I don't need it from you, too. This is my own personal experience of how it all goes down. I'm just a mom with a lot to say. Read it or don't, that choice is up to you.

My hope is that, without judgement, you can indulge in this amateur read and connect with me (and many others) in some random way or form. We, as mothering mammals, should actually try to connect with one another for a short minute, as opposed to engaging in judgement or self-ridicule. That is my hope for this short read.

The sun will rise and then it will set, and The First 100 DAYS will happen somewhere in between.

Female Awesomeness.

For a moment, I would like to pause and reflect and somehow try to wrap my head around this whole pregnancy phenomenon. We, as mammals, are incredible beings capable of something so precious and amazing. Our ability to recreate is a gift, something that should never be taken for granted. God bless our ability to do such a thing, yet my prayers and blessings are also with those who are unable to have this experience. Pregnancy and infant loss and infertility rates are shockingly high, and it is a shame that this misfortune is not talked about on a louder scale. It isn't usually until one has an experience with loss and/or infertility that one learns how common this actually is.

I, myself, have experienced four losses, and I tell you, it's fucking debilitating. It will break you down, but it doesn't have to keep you broken. If you are someone who is suffering with infertility or from pregnancy or infant loss, know that there is help. Please reach out and discover the multiple resources and community that is available to you. People care. Trust me when I say that you are not alone. And as awful as birth and after-birth can be, the inability to create a child and family is much more breaking, and I want that to be very clear while you are reading this book. We make light of the hardship of childbearing, yet we wouldn't give it up for the world. So, remember that when you are crying to the *Kardashians,* or binge eating pails of ice cream in your fat pants – you, my friend, are very blessed. And know that what you have right now, this exact gift, is what someone else is praying for.

Back to mammal talk: The female body is absolutely incredible. Applaud yourself for being able to endure the demanding biological stress of childbirth and the beautiful transformation that our bodies are capable of. Yes, your ass is huge there darlin', and your tits are down to your beltline, but you just grew a tiny human being *inside of your own human body.* From a microscopic sperm, to a full-on human being in less than ten months is a fucking mind-blowing phenomenon. Absolutely incredible. It's a miracle. You. *You* reading this. You put up with morning sickness, the mood swings, the weight gain, the stretch marks, marital arguments, unexplainable anxiety, no alcohol for endless months - not to mention the probability of shitting yourself during labour - all while being stitched up to your ying-yang by a team of hot medical students. All sacrifices which allowed you to create such a precious little baby. (Did I mention no alcohol for endless months at a time?!) Clap those hands, you deserve some recognition for the shit that you've just been through. Applaud yourself. Right now. Do it. I'm serious. Get up. Yell! Scream! Jump! High five yourself! Do it. Seriously. Get up. Yell out loud right now, "YESSSSSSSS" - I just did it in the infamous Oprah Winfrey voice. "YUUUUUUSSSSS!!!" and it felt fucking amazing.

You will probably feel like a bit of a loser, but I'm hoping that your loser self also feels a little bit better. Laugh at yourself. Release is Rhonda. Get up! Jump! Shake those childbearing hips, ya sexy MILF. You owe it to yourself. You just grew a little human inside of your body, and damn right you pushed a watermelon through a fucking pinhole. That shit, right there folks, deserves some bragging rights. They certainly don't hand out medals throughout childbirth or alongside our mothering journey, so do it now. Get up and give yourself some credit. Even if you had a belly birth, a cesarean, never forget what that body was capable of. Own that shit. That's all you, honey, and do not let anyone ever tell you differently. You may feel like an overweight milk machine, because you pretty much are, but you truly are bloody amazing.

As soon as pregnancy, labour, and delivery are over, day number one of postpartum begins. For me, I am using the term 'postpartum' to refer to the days following the delivery of your baby. I understand that postpartum can also refer to a depressive state following childbirth, but for the purposes of this book, I am speaking mainly to the number of days post-delivery.

There truly is no other lifetime experience that will compare to the day that your little one is born. Your life will never truly be the same, for now you have someone else to care for, somebody else who becomes your priority. Your reason for existence and survival has now become the excuse for somebody else. Nothing in life can possibly prepare you for the journey that you are about to embark on, the ups and downs that will frequent your days, and the many times that you will feel lost and alone. No textbook pep talk bullshit can prepare us for the many emotions that will be felt, and the endless number of tears that will be cried. Mostly, we can never possibly be prepared for the amount of love that we could potentially hold for another human being. And, well, let's face it, nothing on this earth can ever prepare us to take an extra hour to pack up the car solely to head around the corner for a fucking carton of milk.

Everything from now on will be a little bit different, will take a little bit longer, and will be accompanied by extra curse words underneath our breath. Forget the razor and your smooth-shaven legs, the skinny brand-name jeans that you will never wear again, and the acrobatic sex positions that once frequented your bedroom. Things will never be the same. They won't, they will just be different. You'll get used to the extra layer of hairy prickles on your legs, you'll have eight different styles of sweatpants for all occasions, and two-minute missionary sex will soon be a predictable norm. Not bad. Just different. And frankly a little bit easier. Never having to shave your legs again? Or get on top for sex? Fuck, doesn't sound like a bad deal after all. Don't believe me? Don't even pretend like you don't change from your baggy basketball man sweatpants to fancier Lulu sweatpants when people come over. It's all about timing and comfort now, ladies. Timing and comfort. And the sex, well, put twelve seconds on the shot clock and call it a night.

Things that were easy now become harder, and things that were once done quickly now take a little bit longer. As tough and demanding as these next 100 days may be, try to remember that you are an amazing, resilient mother, and the naturally imbedded love that you have for your little one *will* get you through this tough time. You will laugh, smile and cry, and will experience moments of true satisfaction and gratitude. You will feel blessed to have created such a cute and wonderful child, but there will be dark days too, filled with pain, guilt, nerves and anxiety. You will experience thoughts and emotional pain that you never knew existed, but always remember that you are not alone. And, hell, think back to the day when broads were having, like, twenty kids with no pain meds. If they could do that, then we can do this. Trust your body. It knows what to do. Chin up, ladies. Slip on those fat shoes (or Crocs, really; Crocs are now your life). Start your engines. Stock that wine cupboard. It's go time.

My female body is fucking awesome because:

_____

_____

_____

_____

My female body is capable of:

_____

_____

_____

_____

Things I have sacrificed are:

_____

_____

_____

_____

Things I am struggling with are:

_____

_____

_____

_____

_____

My favourite pair of sweatpants are:

_____

_____

_____

_____

_____

If I had a ruler right now, my leg hair would be approximately this long:

_____

_____

_____

_____

Birth.

For all us vaginal folk out there - wow. Didn't see that shit comin', did ya? What did y'all think? Seriously. Reading this now after having birthed a child, was it everything you thought it would be? Only you know your story. Which is kinda cool. Only you have that unique birthing journey that is specific to *you*. So, tell me, was it everything that your "birthing plan" was meant to be?

I have heard that those things never go as planned. I have also heard that when we make plans Jesus laughs. If you're not a big Jesus guy, know that what I am referring to is that plans never really work out when we try to make them. Some do, like picking out your nail polish colour at the salon, or binge shopping on Amazon for your own secret Christmas presents, but childbirth? Nah, that shit is hard to predict and will have an even bigger plan of its own. For all of the 'Type A' people reading this without children thinking: *What? Ahhh, I can't plan every single step of how this will go?* No. No you cannot, Brenda. So pop some Ativan or smoke some grass (not if pregnant, obvs.) and get ready to have your hourly day timer put through the shredder because, while we think we have a plan for our birth and how it just might go, it often turns out that our bodies may have a very different plan for us.

This birth and labour thing might look a little different for all of us; like I said, this is your special experience that only you will forever hold. Maybe you started with Braxton

Hicks, which led to contractions and early labour, or maybe you were like me and had your water break before any contractions at all.

During my first pregnancy, I had my water break on my bathroom floor which, in hindsight, was probably the best place for a water breaking situation to happen. Thank Christ it was on my bathroom floor and not in the middle of a Target line-up or, heaven forbid, while I was waiting for my donair to be made earlier that morning. And I must say that I have my sister to maybe partially thank for this. That morning she was telling me to do all the things - ya know, squats, walking upstairs, reaching orgasm. Yes, orgasm (sorry, Dad). I am not trying to be funny or purposely off-side here - it is known that an orgasm or sexual intercourse may have an effect on inducing labour. Try it ladies. I, soon after, went pee to find my mucus plug fall out into the toilet before, seconds later, my water broke. So, thank you sister, it must have been the "lunges" that did it.

I had a huge rush of euphoric energy come over me. Anyone else experience that, too? I recall hopping into the shower to shave my legs and lady bits – if I'm being honest – while jamming to tunes with my mom on speakerphone. I legit had an intense spiritual rush where I was dancing around my house naked. It was awesome, and a bit bizarre, like a legal pregnancy acid hit or some shit. It was good until it wore off. The acid wore off, but my water breaking liquid did not. I think I went through three ginormous pads by the time I arrived to the hospital delivery unit.

That water breaking stuff is some serious shit. For all of those women thinking: *how will I know if it's my water breaking and not just me peeing myself?* You'll know, honey. And I apologize to any women reading this who maybe weren't so lucky. I bet there are a ton of ladies who have had their water break in the line-up at Target.

Whether you start with early labour, or by having your water break and being induced, or with no symptoms at all... whatever. I hope you know what's coming - *the contractions*. Ohhh the contractions. Natural or induced, these motherfuckers are taking over.

A contraction is when our abdomen hardens as it is tightening the top of the uterus. Your abdomen will then soften as the uterus relaxes. This motion of tightening and softening is the process that happens during labour to help move your baby downward. The contractions are what cause your cervix to dilate, or open, making room for the baby to move through it. Contractions let us know that the baby is on its way.

I am assuming you have made your way to the hospital by now. Or, if you are having a home birth, the obvious is that you have called your team of people to come on over and get the party started. The professionals around you will show you to your room, get you undressed, hook you up to machines to monitor vitals and start to prepare you for childbirth and the delivery of your baby.

Word of advice: just ask for the drugs. Contractions can be extremely painful, a pain that is actually indescribable. So, as soon as you get up to the unit, like, while you're checking in, literally just ask for them. "Hi, my name is _____, I'm in labour and I would like all the drugs please." You've gotta, man. I learnt on my first go around - and I'm not sure how it works in other places. When I didn't know how much pain was *too much pain*, they told me that they could not actually *offer* the epidural or any other pain management narcotics, because I had to be the one to request them myself (*something you should probably look into beforehand*). "When the pain gets too bad, just let one of us know."

Fuck, thanks Cindy, I'll just refer to my visual fucking barometer and let you know when my pain tolerance alarm starts to go off. Like, what the actual fuck? This is a stupid fucking rule. When you see me purple in the face, grunting, threatening a divorce with my husband - *offer me the fucking meds*.

When I actually requested them and she 'checked' me down there, well no shit, nine centimetres dilated. *So, Cindy, what you're telling me is that I just underwent six centimetres of enormous pressure and dilation in under an hour without any fucking pain management because I simply didn't know when to ask for them?* My. Fucking. Nerves. I literally wanted to punch her in the vagina. Anyway, fuck. Rule of thumb and my million-dollar advice: call that shit in ahead.

The time will vary between hospital check-in and when you will be in excruciating pain from intense contractions.

Sometimes these are already happening when you arrive at the hospital or birthing centre, and for others having to be induced, it can take time for the contractions to commence. You may have a television to watch, magazines to read, or a stable conversation to be had with your support person. But you're there. Waiting. It's happening. The contractions will soon start to increase in force and occur closer together. This is labouring. You are currently contracting without being ready to 'push' or deliver the baby.

You may receive narcotics or laughing gas *if* you ask for them. An epidural may also be administered, given that it falls within the appropriate time frame. An epidural is a pain medication that is administered into the lower part of your back, freezing the nerves in all the right places. It will allow you to feel numb, alleviating most of the pain that you would normally experience from contractions. Often, women miss the mark on requesting this and it becomes too late to receive the injection. You may be wishing you had called that shit in ahead.

If you don't want an epidural, that's perfectly okay, too. Don't ask for one. Not like you get a medal for that shit either or anything, but it does make for being naked and sweaty while you're panting a little bit more manageable. Your poor partner, trying to empathetically support a giant cat in heat. They're the ones that deserve a fucking medal, putting up with our sweaty mess. Good Lord.

It will make the pushing easier too. I've heard from numerous women, along with little old me, that getting the epidural was life changing. A time where pushing a tiny water buffalo out of your vagina without completely feeling like your legs are being literally ripped from your torso, may actually become possible. It's a beautiful thing. Whoever invented the epidural, you, my master, are a *legend*. No epidural? No problem. I don't care. It's not my vagina. But if that chick is you, I would never, ever want to lift weights next to you at the gym. Your strength and resilience would crush me in, probably, more ways than one.

In some cases, many women wish and request the epidural but are refused because of timelines, accessibility or availability, which can be a damn shame. Let me just say this loud and clear:

If you are a human who has vaginally birthed another human without the use of any epidural or narcotic management – by choice or no choice – you, my friend, might very well be the next prophet.

You are on a different level of heroism. Do you have a biblical name? Like, maybe one that was specifically given to you at birth, destined to be the pain-management-free child birthing Saint of all time? Maybe you were born to do this. I would get my ass to that corner store if I were you and buy some lottery tickets. You, my friend, are one mother-effing badass.

Let's move on from the meds, shall we? Proofreading this I'm starting to crave more laughing gas.

There's a whole team of nurses and professionals in that delivery room, so make sure you utilize them. They've gone to school, they've studied, delivered babies, this is their jam. It's not our jam. I don't want vaginas in my face all day to be my jam. I've got my own jam. I've got raspberry jam and blueberry jam. I don't need their jam. So, let this be theirs. Utilize them, ask them questions, delegate shit, let them help you. You are paralyzed from the tits down, remember? You are going to be needing things. These nurses will be with you throughout your stay here, so let them get to know you a bit. You have endless hours and days ahead of you, and a little supportive help will be very much what you need.

I think I even nicknamed my nurses at one point. Snap-snap. Can I get a bell here? I was polite, don't worry. I have a job, I get the consumer demands, but I was also in a raging lioness state. So, if you were a nurse of mine during the delivery of my first son, then I apologize. I may have had a little bit too much laughing gas that day.

If you are delivering your baby vaginally you will, soon enough, be given the 'go ahead' to start pushing. You have, up until this point, been waiting for your contractions to occur closer and closer together, as well as the opening of your cervix to widen. This is your

29

body's natural way of getting ready for the baby to be able to fit down and out of the birth canal. By now, your nurse has checked your innocent and petrified vagina, and you are dilated enough to where your baby can now begin her journey to the outside world.

Even though we have been under immense distress for hours - contracting and breathing like a dying fucking hyena - as soon as we hear the words *"It's time to start pushing,"* shit actually gets real. There is probably a point for all of us where we think: *"Oh shit, I'm not ready. Nope. I don't wanna do this. Is it too late? Can I back out? How the fuck do I get outta this shit?"* You may start vibrating, shaking with adrenaline. It has never become more real than at this actual point right now. Get ready to be torn in half. Get ready to meet your baby.

You will be asked to put your legs up in the stirrups, the ever-attractive device that allows your legs to spread and your vagina to be spread even wider. This is the moment when we lose all shame. Not only is my husband prohibited from viewing any part of my vagina in the natural daylight, I now have a team of multiple people examining my swollen vagina under some sort of fluorescent fucking strobe light. Feeling overly sexy here ladies? Hang on, it only gets better. And with our luck, the med student is usually always a fucking sexy piece of tail. *Like, really Dr. McDreamy?* Fuck off.

You will push when the nurses tell you to push. If you have had the epidural you will not necessarily feel pain, but you can still feel when the contractions occur. As I requested an epidural for my vaginal delivery, I am unable to touch on what labouring feels like, or doesn't feel like, with the absence of an epidural or any pain medication/management. I am assuming we enter a numb state of shock after a certain pain threshold gives way. I did experience painful contractions prior to the epidural, so I imagine it is something like that, but on illegal steroids.

The contractions you will experience with an epidural are similar to the tightening sensation around your belly that you experienced in early labour, but without the pain. You experience a contraction, or tightening, and then are told to push. You will experience another contraction shortly after and will be told to push again. You can see the contractions on the screen beside you, the little jaggedy thing will fluctuate based on your abdominal and uterine movements. You basically just suffer here until it comes out. So, get comfortable ladies, because I think I was here for multiple fucking hours. I recall my husband being on cold towel forehead duty. He was literally keeping me cool while holding my one leg up as I profusely sweat like a wild animal. God love him, cause I sure as hell don't right now.

I remember pushing, and sweating, and pushing and sweating. But what I also remember is not actually wanting to push *that* hard. I was so worried about shitting myself in front of everyone that I *actually* tried to push from my vagina, as opposed to my ass like they tell you. This might not make sense to those who have not yet had children and that is totally understandable.

I do not expect you to envision shitting the bed when welcoming a baby, but it is just another disgusting thing that we add to our list of *embarrassing items that are completely out of our control*. Usually, when you are giving birth and are in the 'pushing' stage, the nurse will tell you to push from your bum as if you are about to take a poop. *Me? Um. No, thank you.* You might give birth a little bit quicker, but chances are, you will probably shit the bed, too. But whatever. Push hard and get that shit out (literally). Time is of the essence here, and besides, they are all nurses and doctors (and random hot medical students) who have seen it all before. Go ahead, push your ass inside out. What the fuck do they care?

If your baby does not want to break through your vagina in the time frame that the doctor orders, then you may be asked to switch pushing positions. This means altering your body to try to maneuver the baby out of your not-yet-ruined vagina. They may put a padded tri fold thing under your legs to help elevate your uterus and have you try pushing from there. For me, this came with an upper hand bar that I could hold onto as I reached up and pushed, feeling not *just* like a sweating overweight rhinoceros itself, but an *acrobatic* one to boot.

They may also suggest that you lay on your side and experience contractions that way, seeing if baby will shift position by themselves. They will try many things, but I have yet to see a doctor who recommends getting you up out of the bed (with help, of course) and down onto your knees or in a squat-like position. I know what you are thinking, Carol: "This is how I got pregnant in the first place?!" But there's a method to my madness.

Do you think for a second that a pregnant woman who was walking through the woods and suddenly went into labour would actually lay down on her back, put her legs up and expect to give birth to a baby who has to slide up and out in a near vertical motion? No. They would fucking squat. It's simple. Let gravity do its thing. But *no*, we are directed to lay horizontally on a bed and wait for the baby to eventually move in an upward motion, no doubt putting them in danger, until they are all of the way through and out of us. I understand that we are frozen from spinal medication, but let's figure it out, here, *two thousand and twenty*. We put people on moons. Figure out a safe and appropriate way for mammals to act like mammals. It doesn't make sense… *lay on your back and give birth to a baby*. The forest animals are mocking us right now. Fucking idiotic humans. But hey, at least the resident is cute.

You will continue to be told to push and then you will be told to stop. When the baby's head finally arrives at the vaginal opening, you will be told to slow it down. This is a gentle form of pushing that will not tear your vagina any more than it needs to be. This is when your baby makes his initial appearance to the outside. This phase is called the crowning phase.

Not like any royal queen-like crowning sort of stage. Just a head-through-the-vagina crowing sort of stage.

This Way or That Way.

Let's recap: we've had the contractions, the water breaking, the yelling at the partner, the look on our face when we are told that we cannot eat anything for the next twelve hours, the pain meds, the epidural, and the *pushing*. Crowning is when your child's head finally reaches the external point of the vagina: it's almost out.

Even though you may be frozen down there from the heroin-like shot that recently entered your backside, you can still feel most of this disgusting and beautiful experience. I don't quite have words to quite describe the crowning. The initial visual that you see as you push crusty playdough through a small plastic hole kind of resembles the image. Try to have someone snap a picture of it. It's grossly and weirdly actually pretty cool and something that you can revisit, ya know, when you are wanting to reminisce about your vagina stretching to the point of no return. It's disturbing, yes, but also a beautiful part of life's miracle. It's a playdough vagina!

Regardless of the raw image of a somewhat destroyed vaginal opening, your baby has made his appearance.

With gentle hands, and some possible *light* pushing, the doctor will assist the shoulders and rest of the tiny body out of your dilated front bottom. The nurses will then do one of two things: they will either straight-up lift baby directly to your chest, or they will transfer them to the nearby weigh station to get them cleaned off a bit. The first sign of a healthy baby is that initial cry that we first hear. If baby is slow to make any noises, the baby team will assess them at their station.

If you were still unable to push the baby to the vagina naturally within a given time frame, you may be taken in for a cesarean to have the baby safely removed that way. The point is always to get the baby out as safely as possible. Your assigned nurses will be beside you and will be walking you through this the entire time.

Cesarean: a belly birth. Maybe it was planned or maybe it was an emergency operation. I, for one, have had the pleasure of experiencing this fucking crazy thing too. A c-section. Wow. The ability of a team of people to actually cut your body in half to remove another human being is out of this world ridiculous. Think about it. You have a person actually living inside of you, and someone has the ability to cut you open, set all of your organs aside (they literally put my uterus on top of my chest) and remove a baby. Mind. Blown. Pretty fucking crazy if you ask me. The commentary is classic too: "Oh hi there, I'm just putting your bladder over here," or, "now I'm going to put your uterus back together." Like, what type of sick shit is that?

I remember going in for my c-section. I was more worried about my swollen body parts and embarrassed about who might see them, than delivering the actual baby. So, what I did when I went into the operating room was something that I do best, I made a small joke, of course, and trumped my fears with humour. One of the nurses actually replied with an even funnier comment, that being for me not to worry about my swollen vagina, for a recent patient of hers had vagina lips so swollen that she presented looking like two large hotdog sausages. That made me feel a little better. So, I proceeded to demand all the drugs, listening to my own million-dollar advice. I exaggerated my anxiety, nerves, nausea, all of it. Just get a buzz on people, it will go a lot smoother from there, trust me.

One thing about the c-section, and maybe some of you ladies have had a different experience, but whatever happened to just cutting a person open and taking the kid out? This is exactly what a c-section is in theory, but there may possibly be some other hidden sick shit in there too. I'm talking pain, nausea, lots of uncomfortable shit that seems to last forever. I had a high-risk pregnancy with my second and had no choice but to have a scheduled cesarean, so I was kind of looking forward to my vagina staying somewhat intact, not having to shit the bed, etcetera, etcetera. I was also under the impression that they would just simply pop me open like a bag of chips, take the kid out, and stitch me back together.

It was a weird experience, the surreal feeling that even though you are completely paralyzed from the chest down, you have the ability to feel pressure and movement during the entire surgery. I was literally being pulled back and forth, side to side, on the operating table as they tried to pull my son to the outside world. It was very uncomfortable - the tugging, the pressure. And of course, with my luck he was stuck, and a vacuum was needed to assist the process. Trying to vacuum a transverse baby through a complicated cesarean incision deemed difficult. It was painlessly painful. Pretty hard to explain. There was a lot of puking on my end, and even more drug drip requests. There was even more discomfort from the doctor jamming on my intestines as she 'put me back together'. Laying there was a feeling I cannot really find words to describe. I was frozen and couldn't move, yet all I wanted to do was move my feet. I started to feel claustrophobically stuck within myself. The sensation of feeling stuck within my own body was strange and, of course, anxiety ridden. So again, more drugs please.

I'll never forget when they sat me up at the surgery's completion. Looking down and seeing my legs completely spread-eagle, not knowing that they were spread wide open for the entire world to see, was a rather bizarre feeling. Yet, I was too drugged up and exhausted to really give a shit. I, of course, apologized to my husband for any hot-dog like visuals he may have encountered.

Vacuums, suction cups, cone heads - who knows. A diversity of shit can happen during these deliveries. Maybe some women undergo excruciating pain while others are applying mascara at the same time. The experience that we have is unique to us, and no matter the journey, pain level, or amount of times you were denied your narcotic drug demands, you birthed a fucking human.

It's beautiful. And you just did it.

Hello, Baby.

The first time you hold your baby, you will feel an abundance of overwhelming emotions. The many hours of grueling contractions and/or never-ending pushing has finally paid off. Your little one is here. All the anticipation and overwhelming build-up of mixed feelings and anxiety-ridden thought are over. We suddenly forget the painful backaches that accompanied our endless third trimester, and the hangover-like symptoms that accompanied our first. The sweat currently beading off our foreheads and the stale, dry mouth that has caused white paste to accumulate at the sides of our lips doesn't matter in this moment.

Appreciate the human mind's capacity to block out all external stimuli, even momentarily, to forget the last few hours and all of its disgusting moments. Nothing else in the world matters right now. Forget the accumulating mortgage bills, the neglected dog that you left in the backyard when your water broke, or the argument that you had with your partner about what shirt he should have worn for the birth of your little one. It doesn't exist. All you see right now is that perfect little baby. Your baby. You are a mom now. This is day number 1. The countdown from 100 starts now.

Throughout your pregnancy, or at some point within your life, you have probably heard people say that the first time you lay eyes on your little baby it will be love at first sight. That you will immediately and forever be completely and utterly obsessed with your child. Why wouldn't this be the expectation? Every single caption of a new mom's Facebook post is how deeply in love they are. That's wonderful, if it's authentic. We feel pressured, in this day and age, about how our birthing experiences and first moments meeting our baby should look. We all have different journeys and experiences, and for some women, it truly is love at first sight. That is a beautiful thing and a bond that will never be taken away from you. And for some of us, it takes time to build that connection.

In reality, it's like: *uhhh... my swollen kid is purple, just came out with a cone head, and is covered in vag juice*. It takes time for these bursts of life-changing moments to sink in.

I think that we hear things of this nature so often throughout our pregnancy that we naturally build-up anticipation - so badly wanting for those things to be

39

true, believing that they have to be true; that they should be. And they are true, they can be, just not as sugar-coated as all the other 'perfect moms' out there make them appear to be. Try not to focus on how you think you *should*, and are *supposed* to feel when your baby is born. Your emotions and feelings are real. You are scared, nervous and overwhelmed. Give it time. You do love them, more than anything, and once the exhaustion and the initial phases of excitement (and meds) settle for a bit, those feelings will start to become more real.

Do not feel like a bad mother if you are not instantly love-bound to your baby. We've never even met them before, and they are all wet and gunky little alien/stranger people who have just surfaced from a foreign place. You just spent the last how many hours pushing your ass inside out, while profusely sweating, experiencing painful contractions, and most likely ripping your partner a new one. You are exhausted and you probably cannot think rationally, considering all you have been able to consume for the last twelve hours is fucking ice chips. Take a deep breath and shed a couple of tears now, relieved that you can finally get your legs down from the stirrups.

Let the nurse clean off your baby, sit up, take a deep breath, get your shit together, and get ready to start building a relationship with your new little alien. Savour these moments, like when your new baby snuggles into your chest for the first time. It might feel uncomfortable and awkward as shit, and that is perfectly okay. Try not to do anything else but be present. Be still. Breathe. Feel their soft skin against yours. Listen for their breath. Your baby is here.

I say savour the moments because they really won't last long. Not to bring up the truth that, before you know it, your baby will be waving goodbye to you from the bus stop, ready to board the school bus for their very first ride to kindergarten. And in retrospect, after a few short minutes your baby will, no doubt, start crying - screaming, actually. They're probably just cold, tired, hungry, and simply scared shitless after seeing daylight for the first time in their young lives. Everything around them is foreign.

Except for you. Yes, *you*. You and your baby are strangers and you are going to spend the next couple of minutes, days, weeks, and even months trying to get to know each other, but they already know who you are. They know your voice. Your touch. Your smell. Your little babe will feel regulated when close to you, feeling the beat of your heart and the calming aura that they remember from inside the womb. Try to stay calm for them. Breathe for them. Be still. Be present. They need you more than ever in these initial stages. You are their safe place.

Staying calm, I realize, is often more difficult than it sounds. It's stressful in there, trying to bond with your little one amongst the chaos of in and out staff, hospital machines, intercoms, and a husband that left forty-five fucking minutes ago to go purchase you a goddamn Gatorade. Baby aside, trying to sit up comfortably in those hospital beds, with either fresh stitches or an intact catheter, is no joke. (Side note, it's pretty cool that when you have a catheter in you don't *ever* feel the urge to pee.) It's okay for me to tell you to stay calm, because you don't even know me. But when your mother comes to visit and tells you the same, try not to want to rip her face off. (I'll get to visitors shortly.) She's probably just trying to help. Mothers think that repeating the phrase "If you're anxious, the baby can feel that" is helpful. Use your mindfulness skills here and breathe into that baby.

Advice I have for all mothers during these initial hours and first couple of days while still in hospital: don't kill the nurses. You will want to, but I am pretty sure that it will not work out in your favour. They must go through some specific training that brainwashes them to think it's okay *to wake your sleeping fucking baby.* There will be nurses and multiple other forms of humans that flood your room at all hours of the night, often with copious amounts of useless information. The best is the needle poking at 4:00 a.m. and then again at 6:00 a.m. - that's a good one. Or, the paediatrician that needs to come in to assess your little one the moment that they finally fall asleep.

What I enjoyed (*not*) was the nurse that came in to do my med round (you can bet I was buzzing for that shit, on the exact dot of the given hour), and noticed that my eight-hour old son was sleeping ever so cosily in my arms. Even though it was dead silent and three in the fucking morning, she felt it was necessary for my son to sleep in the baby bassinet beside me. Heaven forbid I drop my baby on the floor because I'm so tired and delirious. What this nurse did not know was that I was wide awake and had assistance from my husband to prop up my arms with pillows and cocoon my little boy into a safe and comfortable position, because what's so bad about wanting to hold and snuggle your newborn goddamn fucking baby?

It wasn't very funny when she persisted to move him and un-swaddled him to change his bum once he started crying. He wasn't wet, he was woken up. And no, he's not hungry, he was woken up. And are you kidding me? Is he gassy? No, darlin', you just woke him up. If I knew then what I know now, I would have printed off signs beforehand that read 'Do not disturb', 'Come back later', or 'If we are sleeping, *Fuck Off*'.

They mean well, I guess. So deep breaths, ladies. As much as you want to strangle the next person who comes into your room and interrupts your rest, you'll be back in the comfort of your own home before you know it. Let them do their job. You and your baby are in good hands.

Aftermath.

The physical aftermath of childbirth is nothing but painful and disgusting. That watermelon being pushed through the pinhole that we previously mentioned, well, unless your vagina is made of silky retractable elastic-like bands, don't expect it to look anything like it did before you entered labour. That watermelon did some damage there. I don't care what anybody says, that shit will never be the same. In fact, do yourself a favour and do not, I repeat, *do not* do what every other female does when they arrive home from the hospital and immediately hold a mirror up to your coo-cka. It will devastate you. You will want to divorce your husband.

Truth be told, your vagina has been torn to shreds, and unless you gave birth via cesarean section (which has its own set of physical healing cons), expect to wear a vaginal pad the size of a diaper for the next six to eight weeks. Slap on a name tag that reads 'Granny' and prepare to walk around the house like you would the halls of a nursing home. For the next couple of months, your vagina is foreign. It's old now. It's used. Same with your ass. That whole area in general, it's pretty much a war zone. She'll heal, but like a forest after a hurricane, it'll take time. And by that time, we will be three generations of vaginas deep, so yeah, just accept the state of destruction. Avoid the mirrors. It is now yours to live with.

Don't expect bowel movements to be pleasant. Don't expect there to be any at all, actually. It is quite possible that you will be bunged up for the next couple of weeks. Yes, you read that correctly. A friend of mine didn't shit for *two weeks* after her delivery. I would feel like I hadn't even given birth yet. Gross. And, yes, c-section people this is true for you especially. They have recently frozen your insides, remember, and then had to put you back together after taking you apart. It takes time for those systems to get back to functioning. With the cesarean you are unable to "bear down" on the toilet. So, unless your poop will just slide right out when you sit down on the toilet seat, I suggest you load your cupboard with multiple types of laxatives. That shit's about to be plugged up.

You'll want to pat dry after you use the restroom, or after you and that squirting water bottle share a moment, because, well, stitches. Oh, the stitches. As if sitting in stirrups for hours on end with a whole team of medical staff watching you blow a St. Bernard out of your ass wasn't embarrassing enough, they now have to carefully stitch you back together. How fucking humiliating, but trust me, you really do lose all shame. I think most women will attest to that. That whole lower region just takes a beating after the birth of a child, like a small bomb exploding inside a tiny cave before a respite team comes in to do the clean-up. It's awful. Even more awful is that cave being our most intimate and private possession. On the same token, try not to sweat the embarrassment and

45

the pain - it's short-term. And I bet the medical team working that shift have seen worse - they have always seen worse. Just keep telling yourself that and think of the overly swollen hot dog lady. As for a tip, put a couple of dampened diaper sized pads in the freezer for a while; the coolness will help with vaginal destruction, and for Jesus' sake, ask for more laughing gas. *But ma'am, you've already had the baby, labour is over.* "I don't give a fuck. I'm a paying customer and I want the gas, all of the gas." Requesting to-go bottles might be optional here.

Getting up and out of that hospital bed the next few times, even days, will be a rough go, regardless of the delivery that you had. Don't be surprised if housekeeping has to come in and change the bedding every time you get up to use the restroom. Vagina folk - there will be a lot of blood. But it's okay. That bloodbath created your miracle. You'll be fine. Your body will adjust to childbirth and delivery with endless amounts of bodily fluids and other disgusting stuff.

Even with a belly birth this is true, because your cervix is now open and will still dispense waste to clean itself out. Disgusting, but neat to know that our bodies have the ability to somewhat clean and heal themselves. You've heard that comparison, that your vagina is somewhat similar to a self-cleaning oven. Well, in this case it's more like a self-cleaning industrial chamber. It'll rid all sorts of shit before it's back to its normal self. Ask for a nurse or two, as well as your partner. You will need them to lift your deadweight ass and basically carry you to the toilet. This is where the nurse will spray your vagina clean for you and pat you dry if you wish (we've lost all shame, remember?). They will put you back into bed, only to find you needing to move up onto the pillow another six inches. This, too, will take a team. Your incision will burn as if it's been set on fire and you will cry as if it just split open. The pain is intense. If you've gone this far without any pain meds, I wouldn't hold your breath. You have a help button. Use it.

You will pass clots in the toilet the size of cantaloupes. It's normal, and as the days pass, they will become smaller and smaller. For now, take it easy and accept being bed-ridden for a short while. Get that bell going again. Ring that baby. Delegate. This is your time to be waited on, remember? Put them to work. Your husband, the nurses. You just delivered someone's child, the least they can do is run around the unit stealing muffins or juice boxes from the mini fridge. Demand shit and enjoy it. I took full advantage of the sandwiches in the staff fridges at the end of the hall, just sayin'.

You can attempt getting up and walking around, but if you're not one to enjoy the persistent feeling of your insides wanting to slide their way out as you become vertical, stay put for a while and enjoy the baby snuggles with your new little one. Trust the science of gravity on this one, as well as the catheter. Did I mention that I love catheters?

While trying to quickly heal and gather your bearings before bringing baby home, round up all the free shit you can get. Bring an extra suitcase just to throw stuff in. I'm talking vaginal pads and all the granny panties that go with them. Those hospital underwear are the cat's ass! They are probably the best and most comfortable underwear that you will ever experience in your whole life!! They should make them for men too. Or even just women on the regular; beer drinking Saturdays, buffets, turkey dinners. Breast pads, baby shampoo, blankets, diapers, bottles, even the toilet paper. Hit the fridge at the end of the unit hall; like I said, they are usually stocked with muffins, juice boxes, sandwiches, yogurt. Load it up.

You just provided paychecks for a diverse and extensive medical team, not to mention the unlimited expenses that you now have for the following eighteen years. By all means, stock up. You let people witness and be a part of your very special experience. You just contributed to the economy and local health system as a whole by utilizing their facility and allowing them to gain a new forever-patient. You did your duty of re-populating the earth. So yes, an *I'm entitled to all of this free shit* attitude is warranted here. P.S.- pens. Just for shits. Those health care workers get really worked up when you steal their pens (insert evil laugh here).

Whether your delivery was a c-section belly birth or a vaginal one, your tummy, your legs, your back, your ass, and your breasts will be in pain today, and they will continue to be in discomfort for the next few days - even weeks. Add earlobes and pinky fingers to that list, too. Your body is basically a write-off. It's been detonated, remember? And even though it has been nice stealing free shit from the unit, ordering Skip the Dishes for most meals, and having a holiday from other children at home if you have them, it will be nice to return to the comfort of your own house.

Home Time.

When you get the *a-okay* from your doctor, you will be ready to pack up your belongings, along with all of the free shit you scored, dress your baby for their very first outing, and waddle on out into the real world. Unless you've hired help or have a partner willing to do your dirty work, there will be no one at home to help you wipe your ass, change your soiled bedding, monitor your heart rate, assist in milking your breasts, or spoon feed you Jell-O. You'll have to do all of these things on your own.

So, if you are anything like me, you will hug all the nurses and cry a few tears, as if you were leaving Earth to travel away and live on another planet. It's a weird feeling, having to leave a safe place where you have had your vagina hung out on a clothesline for the last few days, venturing out for your very first time. I never thought the vulnerability of having my lady parts broadcasted to multiple disciplines would equal safety. But in a weird way it did, for me. (I am conscious as I write this, that not everyone may have had a similar experience. If you felt unsafe or mistreated at any time during your birth, delivery, and hospital stay, know that you have a voice and that its okay to advocate for yourself.)

For me, it was surreal walking off the unit with my little one for the first time. I felt like a little lamb wandering off on her own, or a birdie leaving the nest for the first time. Even though I just compared myself to a lamb (it must be the wine), know that I'm speaking to the security and surrounding of professionals that were no longer with me. We quickly forget all of the people over the last couple of days who have seen our vaginal insides and wiped the shit from our ass. It was an oddly safe place to be. And now it's over.

It is a scary thing, becoming a mom for the first time - stepping out into the world as a mother responsible for keeping another human being alive. It's okay, and perfectly normal, to feel resistant and terrified all at the same time. Try to accept these emotions for what they are. Lean into them. Trust in the process. This might be new and scary to us, but the female body has been bearing and adapting to childbirth and motherhood for centuries. Trust in your body that it knows what to do, and trust that your head and heart will follow. We are inexperienced masters of providing maternal care to our little ones. Look how far we've come already. So, take a deep breath, change your vaginal pad for the final time before heading out, and slide those swollen ankles into your shrunken shoes. It's time to take your little one home.

As you waddle your way out, try to remember: you, my lady, are the shit - the mother queen who just created and delivered life. Be proud of that, and, well, hope that your baby will be sound asleep as you load them into the car and embark on their journey back to their first home. I hope you will experience a conscious moment when you walk out of that hospital and think to yourself, *I just had a baby. I did that shit.* I hope you feel more proud of yourself than you ever have before.

You will probably be yelling at your partner to slow down on the freeway, letting every single car pass you along the way. It's terrifying, this brand-new bundle of goodness on a highway for their very first time. I wish calling in police escorts wasn't just a royal thing.

If you happen to be taking public transit home, then feel free to call me for your hero cookie, because that is a whole other level of warrior badass.

The drive home will most likely feel like a long one, as your stitches - both vag-to-ass and cesarean - will feel as if they are burning while unthreading themselves. Count sheep, curse at speeding vehicles, take some deep breaths, and by all means, avoid the potholes.

You're almost home, ladies. Only 99 days to go.

Tip: Throw a Powerade and some five cent candies into your hospital bag. You may also want someone to shoot the images of your baby being born. As gross as it is, we will probably appreciate revisiting those someday.

For that drive home, you may also want to bring a pillow for post c-section care to set on your tummy (the seat belt friction will have you popping all your oxy before you make it home). Or, bring that cold pad for the fresh stitches that hold your female lady parts in place (the one that you would have placed in the freezer earlier on to become an actual 'pad-sicle').

Tip for Dad: If you have a strong stomach, ask the doctor for a visual lowdown on the placenta after it gets delivered. This gross slab of well-done sirloin kept your baby alive for its entire time in the womb. It's actually pretty cool.

My original birth plan was:

_____

_____

_____

_____

_____

_____

_____

_____

_____

_____

_____

_____

_____

_____

What actually fucking happened was:

_____

_____

_____

_____

_____

_____

_____

_____

_____

_____

_____

_____

_____

_____

Things I regret saying during labour are:

_____

_____

_____

_____

_____ is the number of times I requested a drug

drip.

_____ is the number of times I got denied.

_____ is the number of times I puked.

_____ is the number of times I cursed at my

partner.

_____ is the number of times I (embarrassingly

and uncontrollably) shit myself.

Things I would like to apologize to the hospital staff for

are (ie; cleaning up the shitty mess that will leave me

scarred for years):

_____

_____

_____

A prayer I would like to say to my vagina would be:

_____

_____

_____

_____

_____

_____

Personal words of accomplishment for being one of the biggest and baddest bitches around:

_____

_____

_____

_____

_____

_____

_____

The Deets

Vaginal Delivery _____ Belly Birth _____

Pain Management:

Fuck, Yes   _____

No, I am the Hulk   _____

Hospital Name:

_____

_____

Town/City:

_____

_____

Delivered by:

_____

_____

Time of Delivery:

_____

_____

Weight:

_____

Length:

_____

Hair Colour:

_____

Eye Colour:

_____

Hair:

_____

Birthmark:

_____

_____

First Impressions:

_____

_____

_____

_____

_____

Present in the Delivery Room:

_____

_____

_____

_____

First Visitors:

_____

_____

_____

_____

Going Home Outfit:

_____

_____

_____

_____

What we Named You:

_____

_____

_____

_____

Bringing Home Baby.

You are probably both scared and excited to explore your baby's first home. If you are as dorky as the rest of us, you will probably get the selfie stick out to remember that first time on the porch or the initial drive down the lane. Knowing that the baby cannot see more than an inch in front of them, you will probably still tour them around the house. You'll show them their new bedroom and where they will be sleeping, their set up high chair in the kitchen that they won't use until next summer, and your walk-in closet, where they are too young to judge a shopping addiction. You will take them out back and show them the yard, introduce them to their pets, and point over at the neighbour's place. You will walk down the hallways introducing them to random people in picture frames, and will eventually return to your nesting ground, probably your living room or bedroom, where you and your babe will be spending most of your time to come.

You might wonder, in these initial moments, what you are supposed to do with yourself? Or better yet, what it is that you are supposed to do with your baby? *Am I hurting them? Are they sad? Did they get enough to eat?* But the answer is: nothing really. *Keep them alive? How the hell do I do that?* This is as easy and as complicated as it sounds. It's pretty simple in theory: your baby eats, sleeps, and shits. That's all. Yet, it is the most challenging concept of all. It is a routine that will take time to develop, and it's ever so difficult to master with our physical destruction and a peak in our hormones. Be patient here. Bringing home baby is one the of the scariest and most anxiety-ridden things you will ever do. We're here for you.

I hope you left your bags in the car while you waddled your way carefully inside. Your partner will carry those. I also hope you brought that hospital bell home. Your delegation days are far from over. Put that baby of yours in her sleeper chair (that five hundred dollar moon-boom astronaut looking thing in the corner) and plop your ass onto the La-Z-Boy. Get ready to become re-familiarized with Dr. Phil, 'cause ladies: it's you and your tits, the couch, and that baby for the foreseeable future.

From this day to the next, the hours will look quite the same. It will quickly become a cycle that you are familiar with. Feed, diaper change, sleep, repeat. Feed, diaper change, sleep, repeat. Be patient, it will take a while for this cycle to set in and become somewhat predictable. It is all very overwhelming in the moment. We are emotionally distraught, exhausted, and somewhat clueless about what we are supposed to be doing next. Cater to the baby and ride the emotions. It's their world now, we just live in it.

Nurses will have assisted you with housekeeping details and childcare advice before you were discharged from the maternity ward. You will most likely be given sheets from the hospital on which you are to record poops and pees and breastfeeding schedules. You will have been informed of what to watch for and what to expect, as well as healthy vs. unhealthy signs and symptoms, etc.

Some mothers may enjoy these sheets and rely on the information, while others may think they are a complete fucking waste of time. There is an abundance of information, not to mention a list of phone calls to make to your work and unemployment services, but also paperwork to fill out and file regarding birth certificates and SIN numbers as you register your baby as a new human on this earth. As if we don't have a broken vagina already, we have a migraine now, too. There is a lot to think about and at times it all seems so overwhelming. If you have questions or concerns about anything baby related, look to the information provided to you by the hospital. Those contacts are there to support you. Hang in there, an outreach nurse will soon be paying you a visit. And by all means, add paperwork to the list of daddy-duties.

The build-up of anticipation before bringing baby home will have had you placed somewhere along the spectrum of *readiness*.

If you are a very organized and structured person, you most likely have everything in line and ready to go: diapers lined up, blankets and washcloths categorized by colour, nursery perfectly painted and décor aligned. If you are not organized or structured in any sense at all (*meh, all they need is my boob at first*), then that's okay too. Pretty quickly, the bombs will start to go off and newborn outfits will clutter the floor. The laundry will form its piles, the pets will become slightly neglected, and we will all quickly forget the joys of once frequently washing our hair.

Maybe a little bit of mess and imperfection is okay after all. If we are calling a spade a spade here, over-the-top structured women and fly by the seat of their pants women have more in common here than not, don't they? Isn't that what this book is about? Putting aside our differences and insecurities and connecting with the inner experiences that we all share. Realizing that even though we may look and act differently, whether we're structured or unstructured, we as female humans share common ground. Mothers are emotional, hormonal beings and we all birth and raise children despite how organized - or not - we are. *We are more similar than different.*

So, fuck the house mess and the un-returned phone calls. And while you're at it, fuck Instagram and Facebook for a while, too. Disconnect. Wait, what's that? You're bored? Not sure what to do without your Twitter account and endless hours of useless screen time? It's called *Temptation Island* on daytime television. Get used to it. Your new priority is to just snuggle your babe as you pop your oxys, change your granny pad, and clean your vagina with your new squirting water bottle. Get that PVR ready. Netflix is about to become your bitch.

I remember spending a lot of time in my reclining chair. We actually re-arranged the living room furniture for the arrival of the baby. Nesting, as they call it? I was also equipped with endless stacks of blueberry whipped cream waffles, and homemade apple pies. My bathrobe, too, was a hit. A comfortable choice of clothing and easy access to nurse your baby, provided that is the mode of feeding you are choosing. It's about trying to make this new phase of your life easier. So, bring in the new furniture, set up the baby shit, pre-make the lasagnas, get the robes out, whatever it takes. Or not, wing it, whatever. It's a stressful time, so anything to make your coming home days easier, do that. And for the love of Pete, don't forget the laxatives! Trust me, you'll thank me later.

I must say (and I would be curious to know how many women agree with me) that even coming home after giving birth is a strange place to be, emotionally speaking. From a mom of the house point of view, kind of thing. Try and listen to what I am about to say. This might be especially true if we have other children at home:

Because we have just *birthed* a human - vaginal or cesarean, it doesn't matter - our only job is to take care of them and lay on the couch and rest. This is because we are post-surgery/delivery and full of bloody, pussing stitches while being overrun with hormones and exhaustion. Still, we find ourselves feeling guilty for just *sitting around*. Is that just me? Or, is that just me?

It is a difficult place to be, just "laying around" all day, as the world around us continues to move. Even when we are both told, and expected, to stay put and rest there is something inside of us human females, as mothers, that says: "You should be able to do that," or "Cooking dinner isn't that hard," or "I need to go and read to my son, I feel like I'm being lazy." The list goes on. The amount of guilt that accompanies us women as household-together-ers (is that a word?) is shocking, even a day post childbirth.

But as I sit here and write this, I am not sure that I am surprised by the guilt and other emotions that an overwhelmed postpartum crazy lady feels. It all makes complete sense - we should be blown away by a woman's natural strength and resilience.

With every single thing that she has experienced in the last days, let alone months, surviving pregnancy and embracing painful and exhausting childbirth, she comes home exhausted, torn, and broken, only to feel guilty for not doing more. *Wow.* What a fucking weapon. If this is you, ladies (and trust me, a very big part of me was also like *fuck you, I just gave birth to your child. Take the fucking dog out and order me a goddamn pizza!*) then I applaud you. That is a true testament to the woman that you are. You have gone through *so* much and yet still feel obligated, and willing, to step up and fill the powerful role that you hold.

I'm just going to let that sink in for a moment.

I can tell you, most men with fucking papercuts would expect to lay on their couch for a longer period of time, only to watch golf or football because they have a fucking Band-Aid on their finger. You, my stapled-vagina-to-ass lady, are a force to be reckoned with. You will shine throughout your parenting career. Having doubts? Just think about how we handle colds as opposed to the *man flu*.

It may be difficult to put that guilt aside and allow ourselves the rest that we need. Try to prioritize your needs, here. This is an overall short time in the grand scheme of things, and you need to heal your body after the war that it has recently been through. If you have help, utilize it. Mom guilt is a real thing, but our other children in the home are resilient too, and soon enough we will be back up playing with them, giving them all of our draining attention. Be a role model to them. It's a good time to model taking care of ourselves when it is needed the most.

Sleepless Nights.

Your first night will probably be one that you remember. It is your first night as a mother and your baby's first night as your child in their new home. Where to sleep may be a good question? And how? *How am I supposed to sleep with this little baby? Bed? Couch? Do they go in their crib? Bassinet? Shit – we forgot to buy a bassinet…*

Whichever sleeping arrangement it is that you choose, know that this night will quickly come and pass. It will be long in the moment, but it will be a distant memory before long.

For some of us, we have the vision of how these first few nights will go: our baby will be so tiny and cute and will sleep peacefully alongside us in their little cradle as we lay down and stretch our damaged mid parts to get some well-deserved shut-eye until feeding time. When often, in reality, many moms end up sleeping sitting up, one boob out with a cranked neck, just to avoid waking the tiny little beast before they need to be.

You might be that mom who is anxiously awake hearing every little breath and wiggle, or you may also be the kind who passes out quickly from being overly sleep-deprived from the past few days. Whichever one, you will definitely hear your little babe when they awake for feeds, and your motherly instincts will support you with comforting and feeding along the way.

During this first night, while in pain and emotional turmoil, you are their lifeline. They need you. And even if you sit in tears acknowledging that you have no fucking idea what you are doing, know that you are not alone. Know that there are thousands of other women in very similar shoes at this exact moment, thinking that they also have no fucking idea what they are doing. We don't. This is new. But it's going to be okay. Trust your subconscious love and instincts on this. This night will pass, as will the rest. Cranked neck and all, you are doing a great job. Only 98 days to go.

On a side note - and not right away, but when they were a bit older - do you know how much shit I use to get done while nursing at three in the morning? When my kid would feed for thirty to sixty minutes at any given time, I would catch up on paying bills, returning emails, mindless TV, online shopping - the list goes on. Yes, we are wide awake from being sleep deprived and hunched over with back pain while we have a leech attached to our front side. Still, the productivity that occurs during those hours should not be underestimated.

Tip: Load up on TV dinners, snacks, frozen meals, pies, all the calorie-lovin' stuff. You will be hungry. Load up that whole deep freeze. You are now a bear in hibernation. Get your carb pants on. You might find 'coping ahead' helpful here, as well. Set up the hibernation location with pillows and blankets, magazines, laxatives, remote control, phone chargers, mini fridge, whatever it is that you will need to help feel settled in. You will be here for a while.

Bringing home baby I felt:

_____

_____

_____

_____

_____

_____

Thoughts I was experiencing were:

_____

_____

_____

_____

_____

_____

_____

My emotional fucking tornado consisted of:

_____

_____

_____

_____

_____

_____

I had anxiety around:

_____

_____

_____

_____

_____

_____

I was looking forward to:

_____

_____

_____

_____

_____

Pets in the home:

_____

_____

_____

How they responded:

_____

_____

_____

_____

Siblings

Name: _____

Age: _____

Name: _____

Age: _____

Name: _____

Age: _____

Name: _____

Age: _____

Name _____

Age: _____

How they responded:

_____

_____

_____

Our first day together looked a little like this:

_____

_____

_____

_____

My biggest fears were:

_____

_____

_____

_____

Where baby slept their first night:

_____

_____

_____

_____

First night details:

_____

_____

_____

_____

_____

_____

Thoughts/Tips/Notes/Take-aways (i.e. what the fuck have I gotten myself into?):

_____

_____

_____

_____

_____

_____

_____

_____

_____

_____

_____

_____

First night exhaustion rating, on a scale of 1 to 100:

_____

The B Word.

We have other people in our lives outside of ourselves, our babies, and our medical teams. I'm speaking about the F word. Nope, not that one, the other one. Yup, *Family*. I'm also speaking about the B word. No, Darlene. Not that one either. Yup, you got it, *Boundaries*. While not a big deal for some, these can be a really big deal for others.

If you're as blessed as the rest of 'em, you'll probably have the pleasure of your in-laws waiting on the front step at home to greet you. Or your overprotective mother who knows absolutely everything about how to raise a baby. Better yet, a house full of random fucking people because it was somebody's grand idea to throw a little welcome home party for when you arrived.

Please, please, please, have the *visitor* conversation with your partner before your baby comes. This should be included in pregnancy planning from the beginning, so that you have time to drill your wishes into the people around you about what you want and what you do not want. I mentioned earlier that birth plans do not always exactly work out like we hoped they would. Hmmm. Let me reconstruct that. *This* is your new birth plan and the only birth plan that you will need: setting limitations and boundaries around visitors. I wish I could actually be one of those people standing on the corner edge of a ninety-four story tall building screaming from the bottom of my lungs all the way to the fucking mountain tops: *Boundarieeeees, Peeeeople!* They are implemented for a reason and are meant to be respected.

I say tell your partner about these wishes early on, like, even before the positive pee test, because in my opinion, that is one of their main (and only, real) jobs here: setting boundaries and limitations on your behalf. I would, maybe, even get it in writing. Get him to sign it. Print and photocopy multiple copies and have them taped on every wall of the home. I would even slip one into his lunch kit every morning so that he would become somewhat desensitized to the concept. Brainwashing, really.

There can be many mixed emotions and unclear messages on the day that your baby arrives, and at times like these, hard copies with a big *I fucking told you so* stamp will always come in handy. If your partner chooses to allow the unwanted over anyways (perhaps they have issues setting boundaries themselves, or listening and following through on your wishes. Or they simply didn't remember because they, too, are sleep deprived), you have every excuse in the world to let these hormonal colours shine. A divorce is also optional here.

Think about it: you are beyond exhausted, you have just painfully delivered a human being after labouring seemingly to no end, following how many months of anxiety and anticipation, and now the time has finally come to bring baby home and bond together as a new family unit. *Are you really going to want people all up in your home and business?*

Do not feel bad about not wanting visitors during this initial time. I repeat: *DO NOT feel bad about not wanting visitors during this initial time.* Did you hear me? Not sure if ya did there. DO NOT FEEL BAD ABOUT NOT WANTING VISITORS DURING THIS INITIAL TIME.

I should have a homework page attached to this one where you must handwrite one hundred lines of: *I will not feel bad about not wanting visitors during this time. I will not feel bad about not wanting visitors during this time. I will not feel bad about not wanting visitors during this time…*

I do not know why, as a society, we get so worried about hurting other people's feelings. I also don't know why parents feel that they are the exception to this rule. *No, Deloris, you cannot just show up uninvited and do whatever the hell you want for the following however many days. This is my space and I get to decide who is allowed in it. I hear you, you are the mother of my husband, but you are not the mother of this child. Back the eff up and take a number.*

You do not owe anyone an explanation. This is your time. And for fuck's sake, wouldn't it just be nice to sit down in your own living room and whip your boob out without a bunch of people gawking at ya? Enjoy this scary and vulnerable alone time with your partner. You will never get this time back. Bond, and by all means, do not feel like a crazy bitch about it. This is *your* birth plan, nobody else's. Yes, the help may be nice, but the last thing on your mind is the piling dog shit in the back yard or the fact that microwaveable dinners and ordering in will become the norm for the next few days.

Or, who knows, maybe not. Maybe this is a matter of opinion, kinda thing. Maybe it's cultural, maybe these are your own dependent issues, maybe you enjoy people all up in your kitchen in your ugliest and most vulnerable form. Great. I don't know. Request that then. Have your parents over. Have your partner call your friends over. Maybe you want your sister or good friend to be there to support you, or maybe you've hired a doula or maid or private fucking security to help you settle in. I don't know. Whatever. You do you, lady. My point here, and I cannot stress this enough, is do whatever the fuck *you want* and whatever it is that you feel that you need - just please do not feel bad about doing it. These first few days are so crucial and emotionally provoking. So, please, listen to yourself on this one. Trust me: your stretched vagina = your rules.

Over the next few days, people will be harassing you with phone calls, texts, and emails wanting to come meet your adorable new addition. Even though the days are passing, the rule is still the same: you call the shots. The last time I checked, it wasn't anybody else's ruined lady bits. That's all you, honey. If you are nesting and adapting to your new life as a mom by hiding out in the darkness amid the bed sheets, then it's perfectly okay to turn down invitations and leave messages for a later time. Remember that since your partner's genitals were not stretched six ways from Sunday, they are fully equipped and capable of implementing these boundaries themselves. They know how to speak; therefore, they are full-on able to communicate on your behalf.

The opposite is also true. Given that you will want an extra hand or permission to shower this week, ask for help. Get him to do all the texting and phone calling, because trust me, people don't offer it. They might think they do, but it will go something along the lines of: "Let me know if you need anything" or "I'm always here if you need help". *Of course I need help, you fucking moron. I need lots of help.* I may not want people coming and living in my space and messing up my area and hoarding me with useless conversation for hours at a time, but I would sure as shit enjoy a dropped off fucking lasagna, or a text that reads: "I'm coming to take your other kid off your hands for the afternoon, have them ready around two o'clock." So, why don't you just not fucking ask and respond with things that make sense?

You don't see that I just popped out a newborn and probably don't feel like cooking or cleaning, or hey, here's a random self-care package just for shits because my vagina wasn't torn to shreds like yours was. I'll take it. I'll also take a dog walk, a car cleaning, a gift card for food, whatever dude. Because yes, *I need help.* Not sit in my house and stare at me kinda help, but things that would make my day a little bit easier. I swear, people have good intentions, but they don't always use their heads when thinking of the blown apart vag lady.

If you were a smart friend in one of my postpartum days, and I can think of a few, thank you. Thank you for not asking or questioning, rather for simply just showing up. It was meaningful and it was appreciated. So, thank you. For everyone else who 'offered' the help? Like, I love you, but fuck are people a dumb breed.

I remember when my sister texted and said she was coming over to hold the baby just so that I could go shower. Lovely. She didn't say that she was coming over and moving in for four days at a time, nor did she bring a ton of people or dramatic bullshit. She just came, cuddled baby, and left. I had friends who came and left baskets on the front porch, others who brought food and prepared meals. Diapers showed up, as did baby clothes from the neighbours. These things were all very appreciated.

We like to know that we are thought of, without always having the obligation to entertain during this time. I might not have the emotional capacity to communicate with you when my husband is unavailable to fulfil this duty, so by all means people, gain some insight here. Be smarter than the ripped-to-shreds, overweight, milk machine laid out on the recliner. And be okay with when we set boundaries around people overstaying their welcome.

Most people in your circle will be decent about respecting boundaries. Others may not. Please don't be a douche and respect my wishes about who I want in my space. If I say it's not a good time, please don't get offended or take it personally. I have other priorities and responsibilities, some being efforts required to not re-open my stitches as I take a shit or sneeze too hard. Conversing with you might be the last thing on my mind.

Deep breath in, 1-2-3-4, and out, 1-2-3-4.

I remember not wanting to see or speak with anyone for days, even weeks after my second baby, and I remember being totally okay with that. Let's just say, I learned from my first. (You can't tell, can you?!) Set boundaries. Be okay with that. Don't take shit from anyone.

Tip: Have a secret word between you and your partner. It will be a signaling 'code' for when enough is enough, or for when you are past your limit with company. That code word will inform your partner when to implement a boundary, AKA, kick people the fuck out.

Tip for others: Did your friend or family member just have a baby? Ask her partner what is appropriate during this time. Support and provide things that will be helpful - meals, gift cards, diapers, etc., and do not get offended by the fact that it might be more helpful than visiting. Or, be present and available if that is what is needed. Again, check in with their partner. If they are not sure, tell them to ask and figure it the fuck out.

I WILL NOT FEEL BAD ABOUT NOT WANTING VISITORS DURING THIS INITIAL TIME

1 _____

2 _____

3 _____

4 _____

5 _____

6 _____

7 _____

8 _____

9 _____

10 _____

11 _____

12 _____

13 _____

14 _____

15 _____

16 _____

17 _____

18 _____

19 _____

20 _____

21 _____

22 _____

23 _____

24 _____

25 _____

26 _____

27 _____

28 _____

29 _____

30 _____

31 _____

32 _____

33 _____

34 _____

35 _____

36 _____

37 _____

38 _____

39 _____

40 _____

41 _____

42 _____

43 _____

44 _____

45 _____

46 _____

47 _____

48 _____

49 _____

50 _____

51 _____

52 _____

53 _____

54 _____

55 _____

56 _____

57 _____

58 _____

59 _____

60 _____

61 _____

62 _____

63 _____

64 _____

65 _____

66 _____

67 _____

68 _____

69 _____

70 _____

71 _____

72 _____

73 _____

74 _____

75 _____

76 _____

77 _____

78 _____

79 _____

80 _____

81 _____

82 _____

83 _____

84 _____

85 _____

86 _____

87 _____

88 _____

89 _____

90 _____

91 _____

92 _____

93 _____

94 _____

95 _____

96 _____

97 _____

98 _____

99 _____

100 _____

Mandatory Visits.

Oh great, as if we weren't fucking annoyed already, we now have to look somewhat presentable to greet the human who will be judging our motherhood as well as our home environment.

While you are naturally bonding with your baby and getting settled in at home, a mandatory visit with the health nurse is now in order. The best-case scenario for the routine visit, which occurs in the first couple of days after you have arrived home, is having them come to you to assess how your baby is adjusting to life on the outside.

What is not ideal, and what happens often, is you having to pack up and travel to this obligatory health appointment. You know, loading baby back into the car after a solo twenty-fucking-four hours at home, as you bleed from your stitches. All to drive through a snow storm (*Canadians, where you at?*) to be humiliated when asked to remove your top and prove your breastfeeding technique for a room full of fucking strangers to analyze. Here we go again with the shame thing. It's those oversized sausage-like patties that we are very insecure about but feel obligated to display openly to people that we don't even know and feel somewhat uncomfortable with. And yes, I am speaking about those new "mom" nipples.

The nurses and professionals aside, it may be weird even having our partners witness this topless event. For some no, but for some yes. It is a pretty vulnerable place to be, being the only person in the room who is naked and who probably still looks pregnant, while everyone else is somewhat put together, not recently having had their ass split in two, staring back at your naked self. Yeah... that can be a little intimidating and a whole lot uncomfortable.

Your visit will hopefully be short and sweet. They will take your blood pressure, inquire about the baby's poops and pees *(remember those fucking homework recording sheets, because, Lord knows, we have fucking time to record that shit)* and question any other concerns. They, too, will undress your baby, piss them off, and record their vitals. It is either a visit that is a complete disruption and waste of time, or extremely helpful and beneficial in addressing your needs. That is for you to decide.

Visits like these can be overwhelming, for we are still in the hormonal '*I don't know*' stage with mostly everything. The nurses will most likely try to help by giving opinions and offering advice. This may be super helpful, or it may contradict everything that you are currently doing. Remember that it is okay to have different views on what you are doing with your baby. It is okay to feed your baby how you decide you want your baby to be fed: boob, formula, whatever. It's your fucking baby.

Receiving advice and new information can seem like an overload; try and remember to breathe during this time. You really are doing a great job, and you are doing the best that you can.

The nurses will provide input or recommend advice, given there are any concerns with your wee one. They will then leave your home or send you back on your merry way to venture through the snowstorm. This appointment was a great opportunity to address any questions that you may have had. Feel free to request a follow-up visit or inquire about other professionals that you feel you may benefit from contact with, like a lactation consultant, for example.

As much as the help and assistance is nice, it can be hard to tolerate other people during this emotional time. We are stressed out and we are tired, so know that irritability is flying high here, ladies. Hopefully, you'll have been given pamphlets and different resources on what accessing help could look like. There are a variety of areas that could require focus during this time: sleep, nutrition, breastfeeding, social connection, and mental health support, just to name a few. Know that help is available to you and know that during this time it is okay to ask for what you need.

We've been doing a lot of breathing in this book, so just remember that breathing is a skill that we may need during this appointment, along with other appointments that you may have, such as breastfeeding consultations, pediatric meetings, cosmetic procedures, new moms groups, etcetera.

Breathing is a skill that we are about to master.

Tip: Seek more narcotics. Just kidding. Or am I? Take this time to utilize the resources that are in front of you. Ask questions, seek clarity. Even if you do not have specific questions or concerns at this time, ask about contact numbers that could come in handy on a later day. Chances are, you may need them.

Questions:

1 _____

2 _____

3 _____

4 _____

5 _____

Notes:

_____

_____

_____

_____

_____

_____

_____

_____

Name of current narcotics (You may want to remember these so you can call that shit in ahead for next time):

_____

Resources:

Name: _____

Phone Number: _____

Service: _____

_____

Name: _____

Phone Number: _____

Service: _____

_____

Name: _____

Phone Number: _____

Service: _____

_____

Name: _____

Phone Number: _____

Service: _____

_____

Name: _____

Phone Number: _____

Service: _____

_____

Name: _____

Phone Number: _____

Service: _____

_____

Name: _____

Phone Number: _____

Service: _____

_____

Name: _____

Phone Number: _____

Service: _____

_____

Name: _____

Phone Number: _____

Service: _____

_____

Milk Machines.

The first few days at home are especially difficult and overly intense because, not only do we have to meet with unwanted nurses and fill out endless amounts of overwhelming paperwork, we are pretty much cows who have to figure out appropriate ways of extracting milk from our utters, or have our infant survive from another feeding method. Even writing this sentence, having breastfed two boys, the last one off the boob about three months ago, it still gives me anxiety thinking about that critical time. For me, this was one of my most significant struggles, one that persisted until the day I finished nursing, actually.

Feeding is something that will constantly change as your milk supply changes, as the baby grows and develops, as their preferences change, as bottles, and pumped milk, and babysitters, and nipple shields, and hormones, and wine nights, and many other things all come into play. *Fuck.* Would it be rude if I actually just left this topic here and moved on to a different one? It is stressing me out already. How do I even talk about this diverse topic without confusing the people reading this who haven't had children yet? Well, let's just start by saying: it's a complicated one. Here goes my best shot at a breakdown of this whole breastfeeding thing, and please try your best not to judge me for it: You will either breastfeed your baby or you will bottle feed your baby. You may even do both. That's all. K, bye.

Kidding.

Breastfeeding your baby means that they will suck on your nipples, extracting milk that you naturally produce as a mammal. Which is why I refer to us women as cows, in a very soft and genuine way, of course. Maybe that's why I even felt like a lamb earlier? Are lambs mammals, too? Anyway, in theory, you will nurse your baby on one boob, burp them, and then give them "dessert" on the other. At the next feed, two to three hours later, you will nurse with the boob that you left off on, and then finish with the other. You rotate boobs. This is to even out milk supply. The more your baby eats from one breast, the more it will produce. Supply and demand here, folks. So, even out those puppies. If you do not, and you mainly nurse your baby from one dominant side, then one boob will be a Yorkie and the other will be an English Mastiff.

I said that the next feed would be about two to three hours later. Well, cluster feeding is also a thing where babies pretty well nurse around the clock. Not fun times, but it does happen.

A bottle-fed baby means that your baby will feed from a bottle, as opposed to your breast. Formula is typically used for bottle-fed babies, either as a personal choice, or when women are unable to naturally produce enough milk.

Breast milk is also used to bottle-feed babies. Babies may have health-related concerns which do not allow them to suck successfully from your nipple. They may also not prefer it.

If a mother still prefers to feed their baby with her breast milk, she can do so via a breast pump and bottle.

Women may "pump" the milk out of their breasts using a breast pump, very similar to the machine that manually connects to the cow's udders on a dairy farm. A breast pump is a man-made machine that allows milk to be manually extracted from your breasts. The milk collected will then be fed to your baby via a bottle.

There are many reasons why women may use a breast pump, aside from it being the primary manner of feeding their baby. A woman may pump if she misses a feed and becomes engorged or when these little bastards get picky and refuse one breast altogether. Pumping is used to even out breast production (remembering the yorkie and the mastiff).

A woman may also pump to have extra milk for storage.

I, for one, have always enjoyed my wine. So, I always preferred to have extra milk in my fridge at all times in case it rained and I needed a drink.

Pumping is a lot of work. I was lucky enough to naturally produce a plethora of milk with both of my babies, but some women are not so fortunate. Some women find themselves pumping every few hours around the clock, for months, just to maintain supply. This is a whole other level of exhaustion and commitment. Women will pump regularly when they feel their supply is decreasing prematurely - the more we pump, the more we produce.

I would sometimes pump after the baby had "dessert", storing that extra milk in the freezer. It adds up quickly and can come in handy on those days when you are unable to make it home in time for a feed or have childless commitments outside of the home. *And* also, on those days when you get "stuck in traffic". (AKA met your girlfriend for a long overdue cocktail on the way home from a shopping spree on your secret credit card.)

Educate yourself on freezing and storing breast milk if you'd like. Pumping is a great way to ensure that you have extra on hand if you ever need it. If you didn't feel like a cow before, stand in your kitchen topless with the breast bump connected and crank that puppy up. Your utters will be out in full bloom. And if your partner still loves you then, along with having seen what your vagina did in that delivery room, you guys can get through pretty much anything. But I still might sign the prenup.

Easy, right? Sure, in theory. Those little bastards can get picky though, sometimes refusing one breast altogether. Yeah, crazy right? *It's food, ya beautiful little jackass. Just eat it.* Your breasts will quickly tell you if they are not being nursed from, as those bad boys have a mind of their own. You will feel the pain as your breasts fill up and you become engorged (swollen) with milk. You will need to extract this milk, so hand pumping or using a breast pump is necessary here. The feeling of engorgement can be extremely painful. There are things you can do to help soothe the process, such as warm/cold washcloths or massages.

Blocked ducts are a thing too - this means that one of your breast ducts, or pathways, is clogged and the milk is unable to flow freely to the nipple. You may be able to see and/or feel lump-like areas of tissue. This can be extremely painful and may even require medical attention if soothing techniques do not provide relief or resolve the issue.

The stressful part about nursing/feeding is that it isn't always smooth sailing, if you couldn't tell that by now. We often have to teach our little ones how to eat. Perhaps they were born with a tongue tie, aversions, or were born prematurely and have not yet developed their sucking reflex. These things can take time and medical attention and are more stressful when we are so sleep deprived.

What's super fucking annoying is other women's advice around how you should or shouldn't be nursing your child. The best advice can be from people who don't even have fucking children. *I literally bit my tongue when writing that sentence.* While we are currently lacking the ability to function and communicate with others, we are mostly lacking the skill of patience. If trying to connect with, and train, a crying stranger is not stressful enough, the last thing we need is a bunch of comments and suggestive advice from kidless fucking single ladies. If that is not shoot-me-in-the-face fucking annoying, then I don't know what is. I kind of wish I had one of those invisible dog collar things and I could magically put it around people's necks, and every time something idiotic came out of their mouths I could just give them a little zap. Fuckers.

Here may actually be the best and smartest tip of this whole book. I may suggest getting it tattooed on your forehead:

No matter what idiotic advice you receive,
or how defeated you feel,

Do Not Give Up.

This is a learning curve and it will soon figure itself out. You know your stranger the best. As a team, you two will get it sorted. It will all be okay.

The demands of producing milk, as well as formula feeding around the clock, can certainly exhaust our capacity to manage emotions. Again, this was one of my most stressful times in the beginning stages. *Are they getting enough milk? Are they intaking too much air? Are they peeing? Gaining weight? Why won't they eat? Why are they fussy? I'm so fucking tired I don't want to get up and pump! And holy fuck, my nipples hurt.*

It is a time where we will most likely feel defeated, guilty and scared. A time that truly does take a toll on our overall mental health. We feel pressure to produce adequate milk and assist in our young stranger's survival. It is a never-ending form of exhaustion that just "comes with the territory". No matter how defeated you feel, know that throughout this struggle to manage and figure this all out, and despite the frustrations you feel through your tears, you're doing it. You are actually doing it. It's a struggle, but you are pumping and nursing and feeding and pumping, and you are *doing it*. Your baby is alive and all you can do is continue to try without giving up. Power through. Keep going. Don't give up. I've said it before and I'll say it again: it may not feel like it in the moment, but you're doing a great job.

Breastfeeding is complicated because many women want to nurse their babies naturally, but cannot. Or, their supply is there, but not in full. Or, women have a large supply, but their baby will not take the boob. Or, their supply has suddenly decreased and they now have to supplement. But their baby won't take a bottle nipple because it is used to a regular nipple. But not a *regular* nipple because it was actually using a fucking *nipple shield*. So, now this baby is suddenly on a hunger strike and won't take any fucking nipples. And they are up screaming and distressed because they hate all nipples, but all they really need is just *any* fucking goddamn nipple. And you are stressed out because you are becoming engorged, and your tits hurt, and you've wasted too many dollars on different formula and an array of random fucking nipples just to try to get your baby to fucking eat. *And why won't they just fucking take a goddamn fucking nipple?*

Breathe…

Sometimes they love the boob, the next day they don't. They are possessive little creatures who will take the formula bottle one day, and then gag at the same damn bottle the next. It is a goddamn fucking coin toss. They have no idea what they actually want. It's pure chaos. It's gambling with monsters. They are like these argumentative little dictators refusing food intake. It's like seeing a poster board with people on strike, and one side is an overly sized angry Russian mob protesting to protect their political rights, and the other is a fucking baby reading "I won't drink milk." *You're a week old, calm down there, Slim Shady. What the fuck? Just take the goddamn fucking bottle.*

Yes, feeding children can be very stressful. Breastfeeding, bottle feeding, fucking pump feeding… it's a little bit of fucked up and a whole lot of crazy.

So, super stressful, yes, but another freakin' miracle. Am I done here yet? Any more questions? Good, don't call me.

Even with all of the above circus show chaos, the mind-fucking stressors involved with figuring out how to actually keep a five-pound human alive (or twelve pound, sorry Alma and your vagina) can truly be pretty amazing. The ability to naturally excrete milk from our body - that is amazing - not to go all 'science' on you or anything. Wanna know what else is amazing? The amount of milk we are actually able to produce. Whether we struggle to produce small amounts of milk, if any, or we can pump a crazy eight ounces at any given time, we make milk - and good milk. Not government regulated, hormone added, sugar infested, white Pepsi kind of milk. We make *milk*. If you add up all of that milk, produced and extracted exclusively from nursing mothers on a global scale, well, the dairy industry should be borderline threatened by us.

Again, we are a force to be reckoned with.

Your breast size will enhance during this time, as it did throughout your pregnancy. Some women like and take pride in that; the only probable time where they can feel like Dolly Parton without having to pay what some women pay to go under the knife for. You will see an expansion in these bad boys when your milk initially comes in. This takes a day or two after the delivery of your baby. They may seem as if they will actually burst open, and the veins that cover them will look like directionless road maps. They might look great, like the boobs that you never had (they're not deflated yet), but they will leak and bleed and do all sorts of sick and scary shit. Buy some nipple pad cover things if you feel the need. Paper towel works well, too.

Both breastfeeding and bottle feeding will definitely take some time to figure out. You will no doubt struggle through these next few days, in particular. Hang in there. It's a rough go. You're doing the best that you know how to do.

And that is good enough.

Tip: If you are having difficulty with getting your baby to latch (often prematurity or tongue ties can influence their ability), then inquire about a nipple shield or look for one at your local pharmacy. This is a great tool that women do not always know about. Lactation consultants are a godsend. You may have encountered one already. Let them be your bible.

My boobs used to:

_____

_____

_____

_____

_____

They now fucking remind me of:

_____

_____

_____

_____

If I had a name for my long-lost breasts, it would be:

_____

_____

_____

_____

One of the biggest nursing/feeding struggles I had was:

_____

_____

_____

_____

_____

_____

_____

I have written a letter to my breast pump, and it is this:

_____

_____

_____

_____

_____

_____

_____

Nipples.

Oh hiiiiii, sausage patties, when did you get to town? Did we talk about nipples yet? Like, of course we just talked about the breastfeeding, enlarged boobs and blocked duct kind of nipples, but did we talk about the actual *nipples*? I'm speaking about those now-foreign objects that currently dangle from below your neck. Haven't noticed? Good girl, I was going to suggest not looking down for a while.

I hope you are not analyzing those boob charts that swarm social media, trying to figure out which boob 'n' titty pic best resembles your new rack (but don't act like you haven't *actually* looked for it). During pregnancy, you no doubt watched those nipples expand and morph into the darker, pancake-like saucers that we see today. We might despise them and think they are unattractive, but just like everything else, they serve a purpose. These hormone-ridden bodily changes upon our breasts actually help our young ones navigate to their food source; they are drawn to the darkness. It may not be pleasant, but it is nature's way of sustaining our offspring.

I'm hoping you were able to jack some nipple cream from that hospital unit of yours, because Jesus knows, you're going to need it. Whether you are breastfeeding your baby or not, you probably attempted to in hospital, solely for the initial colostrum that is beneficial to your baby. Your boobs will hurt, regardless. Either from breastfeeding (yes, they will most likely crack and bleed), from pumping (yes, they will mostly likely crack and bleed), or from not breastfeeding and having to endure the unavoidable pain of your milk engorging your breasts (yes, they will feel as if they are probably going to crack and bleed).

If you are nursing your baby in this initial stage, you will experience the raw adventure of cracked nipples. They are not used to being forcefully sucked on for hours at a time, and just like anything else, they will respond to that. They will develop open sores and become chapped and bloody, only to be fed from moments later by the same hungry, toothless predator. We have no choice but to endure the suffering, for the lives of our helpless creatures depend on it.

Your nipples have grown and changed, and are feeding your baby now. They are swollen, cracked, bleeding and sore. I'd like to think of them as a newly purchased pair of converse shoes. Yeah, I can just feel the ladies nodding their heads at this one. Converse shoes are a *bitch* - until you break them in. They take time. Your heels might bleed and become swollen, you may even develop calluses on the sides of your toes. But your feet are simply adjusting to the stylish new way of walking that has been presented to them; they will adjust in time. So, keep going. Don't give up. Your feet will adjust to the overpriced shoes, as will your nipples to the mini hungry tiger/piranha. Use the nipple cream, let out some tears, and, by all means, curse your husband's name. You will get through this, one nipple cream ChapStick at a time. (You can overuse it, too, it's not a narcotic.) Carry on forward with your night. The calluses will eventually establish themselves, and the sun will soon rise again.

Power through these first few days. It will not take long until these bad boys adjust to the hangry little munchkin who is obsessed with them.

You got this.

Aaaaannd that's a wrap on boobs.

Seriously.

For real.

I'm done.

I never want to see another fucking nipple in my entire life again.

Tip: Nipple cream, cold and warm compresses, no self-judgement.

If my old nipples had an obituary it would read:

_____

_____

_____

_____

_____

_____

_____

_____

_____

_____

_____

_____

_____

Mood Stuff.

The physical aftermath of surviving a bloody war zone, disrespected boundaries, mandatory medical appointments and the impossible task of figuring out a painless nipple feed are all things that can leave a woman feeling heavily defeated. Not only is childbirth a chemical transformation in itself, many other outside factors contribute to the overall demonstration of a Wednesday night circus show.

Single lady with no kids: not sure what a fucking chaotic Wednesday night circus show actually fucking looks like? Go grab a random partner who you only like half of the fucking time…

… then borrow a screaming baby for the evening, rent a yappy chihuahua, rip open your abdomen just for fun, throw in the neighbour's toddler or two just for shits, attempt to cook dinner for the entire family while breastfeeding and pumping raw, cracked nipples on the side. Meanwhile, try to build train sets and read books and build LEGO and pour baths while still catering to a crying baby and whiny siblings. Fold the laundry, clean dirty toilets, and please your endlessly horny rented husband. Oh, and by the way – *keep your fucking shit together*.

It is a burden that is heavy to carry.

It is not voluntary. It is expected.

It is heavy. It is hard. It is challenging. And with support, we will survive it.

Chemical Stuff.

When a woman gives birth there is a dramatic drop in her hormone levels. Think about it. We are growing a human inside of us; from a microscopic organism to a full-sized infant in a number of months. When that human is physically detached from our body, from blood lines, cell formations and bodily pathways, there is a significant chemical transformation that occurs within us. The sudden drop in hormone levels can activate and intensify mood swings, and the hormonal fluctuations, mixed with many other psychosocial changes such as exhaustion and fatigue, can leave a woman feeling highly disconnected and overwhelmed. The collision of these things sits heavy on a new mom and her ability to function at a somewhat tolerable level.

The kicker? She isn't allowed to give up, she is not allowed to simply 'take a rain check' or disappear under her bed sheets for the coming months binge watching Shameless (although how fucking awesome would that be?). She isn't allowed to call in sick or show up late to life or transfer all responsibilities onto her partner. She is forced to power through. She has a dependant now who needs nurturing and feeding in order to survive. So, she will bear the chemical hindrance and perform her motherly duties, all while in a fog of fatigue and exhaustion.

Seems fucking crazy, doesn't it? I don't even feel physically capable of keeping *myself* alive right now - literally. I'm over here surviving only on water, oxys and laxatives, but now I have to keep someone else alive? Yes. Oh, and while you're doing that foggy, depressed, teary eyed, overwhelmed, bleeding, popping hemorrhoids, constipated, and a bit high on drugs, will you please record and fill out these pee and poop charts, monitor for jaundice, analyze your own blood clotting size chart, and then drive through the snowstorm to report to one of us nurses? Don't forget to be prepared to show us how efficiently you can breastfeed your child so that you don't have to return in the following days for weighing, measurements and vital analysis (sorry, I'm still not over that).

Oh my God. I can't even.

We go through so much. It's no fucking doubt we want to throw our husbands out of the goddamn window most of the time. We are fucked up. This shit is real, and often very out of our control. The low mood, the fluctuation in hormonal levels, the mood swings, the gratitude, the crying, the zoning out, the anxiety, the anticipation, the love, the exhaustion… And to think that as we have to cope with all of this, keeping our head above water, we also feel physically disgusted and depressed with the foreign body we see in the mirror. It's a lot; the physical and emotional toll. Who the hell are we? It is hard to manage. We feel alone, isolated and like nobody understands. Perhaps we even self-isolate, as a way to unconsciously protect ourselves. *No one can see me like this. No one wants to see me like this. Nobody gets it - I'm all alone.*

They say that day number three is the hardest and most challenging, in terms of the imbalances with our hormones. On this day, and many others like it, you will no doubt cry at the dinner table for no reason, become irritable to the point where even *you* know that you're being a bitch, and you will find yourself uncontrollably sobbing and snapping for no reason at all. This is all normal. This is expected. This day is the peak.

We often feel like we won't get through the unexplainable rush of emotional distress, but by some God-given miracle, we do. We get through that third day, we get through the next, and we survive that first week. As we do, from day to day, we notice that those hormonal levels tend to shift a little bit more every day. The irritability lessens slightly, and the resentment becomes a little less jagged.

We are women going through the motions. We are tired, but we are also resilient. We are strong. We are warriors. We will power through.

This is week one.

Mom Bods.

Our new bodies will impact our mood. Whether it's our boobs and new-neighbour nipples, the extra pounds we have recently added on, our vaginas being raw and freshly stitched, or our c-section incision that has recently been stapled together; childbirth has taken an immense physical toll on our female bodies. We were stretched and then opened, and then put back together again. We might as well sit on a fucking wall and have a great fucking fall while painfully reciting: *Humpty Dumpty had a big baby, Humpty Dumpty had a big tear, all the cute nurses and doctor men, couldn't save Humpty's vagina again. (Pours another glass of wine.)*

We often consider ourselves used and damaged, and why wouldn't we? We have been through unexplainable turmoil.

We have gone from a 'before' body to a now foreign fucking Humpty Dumpty bod that is staring back at us. Our hips are wider, our tummy is flabbier, areas are invaded with stretch marks, even our feet have fucking grown a size. This body is different, it's weird; chances are, we are finding it difficult to connect with. Body image, ladies - this will bring many of us down.

We grieve the loss of the physical person that we once were. But on the other hand, our current body may not be one that we hate completely. In fact, we may hold high respect for our newfound body. It has recently done incredible things. We should be grateful for that. But just because we understand the ever-changing bodily formation of a childbearing woman does not mean that we have to be *okay with it*. We can respect our body and still feel saddened by its transformation. It *is* possible to appreciate our body and feel defeated by it at the same time. It *is* okay to feel lost within our own skin; knowing that our body just did a beautiful thing while feeling simultaneously unsatisfied with the result. This *is* a big change. This *is* foreign. This *is* uncomfortable. This *is* normal.

This is us undergoing the effects of creating another human being. It's not supposed to sound appealing - and again, we do not have to be okay with the reality of an evolved body shape - but that body shape produced a human. It has done incredible things. Miracle things.

Our human body itself is the *only* physical thing in this entire world that we will *ever truly own*, and it has recently been transformed almost beyond recognition. Carrying and birthing children is a huge change. It takes a significant toll on our overall sense of self and the way that we perceive who we are. We may look into the mirror and hate who we see. We may often feel like we do not recognize or connect with the image staring back at us. We may cry, seeing what our body has morphed into. We may become angry at what pregnancy has done to us.

Feeling defeated by our own body is a darkened state that leaves us feeling hopeless and like strangers to ourselves. In these days following childbirth, with emotions running high, it is difficult to be optimistic and rational in the thoughts we have around Self. Our already depressed outlook has us viewing most things, especially our bodies, in a negative light. It may be challenging in the moment, but trying to be kind and compassionate with yourself might be the token that gets us through each day. If you have a trusting and optimistic person in your life who understands all of this, reach out. Their advice may be the countering rationale that you need during this time.

We tend to look at having children as being an overly positive experience. We glorify pregnancy and the ability to capture a picture-perfect family photo. We tend to speak about the good things that happen like the cute laugh and giggles and how fortunate we are to have been able to carry a cute little baby to term. We look at trips and milestones and hunky-dory fuckin' Saturday luncheons. But behind the smile and the private door of our home, it tends to be a darker place at times. One that's not often shared or announced, and not usually broadcasted over social media in a genuine manner.

Through the blood loss, the pain, the surgeries, the stitches, the stretch marks, and the surreal feeling of seeing our body undergo so many changes during the many stages of pregnancy and childbirth, the physical transformation is only the surface. What happens underneath all of that is so much more.

Isolation.

Staying at home with a baby is a very lonely time. It is a drastic change, going from regular socialization to sitting on the floor for three hours at a time with nothing but a baby to entertain you. Fuck. The under-stimulation that I felt was depressing in itself. I recall having no one to talk to, no one to call, and no one to simply connect with on a daily basis. I became irritable quickly and would get easily frustrated when the baby acted like 'a baby'. I began to resent him. He was the beautiful accident that interrupted my life, halted my education, and distanced me from my peers.

Staying at home with a baby will be overwhelming in its demands, yet boring in its social opportunities. After the novelty of meeting your new baby wears off, your phone will be quick to silence and your work email inbox will soon block you out as being unavailable. The neighbours will carry on with their daily routines and life outside of your four walls will quickly forget about you. It's funny how quickly people in your circle distance themselves, retreating back to their own lives. Not that they selfishly mean to, but as a natural consequence of having their own lives and shit going on. "Hey, I met your baby and brought you a present, now I'm going to fall off the face of the earth and not text you for the next six months." *Great, thanks Paula. Way to make a girl feel loved.*

People have their own shit going on - they don't think to reach out and text and connect with how you and your own depressive life are doing. And when they do, it's all about the baby: *How is the baby doing? How is the baby eating and sleeping?* No questions are usually posed our way about how *we* are actually doing, eating, sleeping, and functioning. And besides, these are things that are not always talked about, so why would people know to think about how we are feeling and if we are depressed and super isolated? They don't. They have their own lives. And that's totally okay. We should be happy for those people that they have so many other reasons in their own lives to be busy. Truly. It just makes our new life and world a little bit lonelier.

Maternity leave and motherhood are isolating. It is perhaps one of the loneliest times in a female's lifespan. (That is not credited, I totally just made that up. But I am super sure that it actually is.) When else are we this fucking lonely? When our high school boyfriend breaks up with us after six months of dating? Boo-hoo. Go smoke a joint and get a random number from some guy at the bar. This is a type of loneliness that's on another level. It's *emotionally* lonely. Not the breakup type where were feel like someone left us and we are heartbroken because we feel like our lives are over forever. It's much darker than that. It's to a depth that leaves us feeling darkened all the way to our core. We are in such a zone that the disconnection we experience has us shattered within our own existence. We are blurred with blackness and defeated by our own inner self talk. Our world gets small. It gets quiet, but at the same time, a lot louder. We become depressed. We become distant. We become isolated.

Depression and Anxiety.

These are both very real things. The introduction of a new baby can impact our mood significantly. Those chemical changes and hormone fluctuations that we previously mentioned can leave us feeling low and with unwanted thoughts about ourselves and our babies.

It is normal to feel low and saddened due to the circumstances and the hormones. Women often experience postpartum 'baby blues', which include mood swings and moments of crying. These bouts of low mood will begin soon after childbirth and will typically last the first couple of weeks after arriving home. For some women, the duration of this depressive state is more severe and lasts longer. Here, women might feel tired most of the time, cry more excessively, have increased irritability, fear, hopelessness and the inability to be present and concentrate. Furthermore, women may find it difficult to bond with their wee one - they may not even want to spend time with their baby at all. Becoming withdrawn and experiencing some pretty crazy, intrusive thoughts can be pretty common.

Anxiety is something that a lot of women also experience post-birth. Anxiety often leaves us feeling overwhelmed, facing unwanted thoughts and endless worry. We can often find it difficult to calm our minds and so become irritable and on edge as a result. We may see changes in sleeping and eating patterns. Women may also experience physical symptoms within their bodies such as sweating, shaking and heart palpitations. Panic attacks could be experienced.

All of these symptoms can be normal, of course, but they can also be very dangerous and life threatening when severe and prolonged. We may think that we are able to handle it or that we are *supposed* to be able to handle it. Know that it's okay not to have it all together all the time. Please know that it's even more acceptable to ask for help. Seek feedback from your loved ones, and try to listen to their concerns if voiced. Many of us cannot objectively view our behaviour when we are 'in' those moments. Try and be honest with yourself. You know yourself the best. If you feel like something is off, if you feel like you cannot manage anymore, if you feel like you should reach out for help, you probably should. We are warriors, but even warriors can benefit from help at times. There is strength in acknowledging our challenges.

Note that anxiety and depression can occur at any stage, often first appearing during pregnancy itself for some women. These symptoms can last until your child's first birthday, or, may even occur periodically throughout your life due to external and circumstantial events.

When I had my first son, I can honestly say that I cried every single day for about three months. I didn't know why I was crying at the time, I just remember sitting on the couch with my wee one and as he cried, so would I. I felt sad, and so I would bawl and ugly cry. I just felt overwhelmed. It was when I was alone with him that I would sit with too many of my thoughts, or perhaps when I didn't have any thoughts at all. I was disconnected from my work team and from my other friends who didn't yet have children. It was very isolating at times and was difficult to feel alone.

Even though I was overly emotional and slightly depressed, I felt so grateful to have a perfectly healthy baby. I would feel a whole mix of shit. I would feel alone, but feel grateful; and feel sad, yet fortunate. I was happy to have a child, yet I felt torn from my independence. I was angry at times, feeling robbed of certain things. I was jealous of others and angry that it wasn't something that I had been able to plan. I was sad, but mad, but happy, but depressed, but grateful, but annoyed, but so very thankful. It was a hurricane of spinning emotions, not knowing how to cope with all of them at once. I bounced back and forth and often felt alone. I believed no one would ever understand what I was going through, that it was just me who felt this way.

It wasn't just me. I thought it was just me, but it wasn't. It was me, sitting and crying in my house all alone, like every other mom out there who exists after childbirth.

You are never crying alone, per se. You are crying and feeling alone together with thousands of other women crying and feeling alone at any given time.

Minutes will pass, and hours will quickly turn into days. The exhaustion that persists will become a blur that will literally carry you from day to day. Your life will seem boring and routine, but also emotionally demanding as you continue to struggle with feeding around the clock, and balancing your home life, other children, and social relationships on the side. Figure out that breastfeeding pump bullshit, ride out the hormones, eat all the pizza, ask for help if you need it, and couch like you have never couched before. How long have you been home now? A week? Hang in there. Only 93 days to go.

As the days and weeks pass, things will hopefully begin to level out - hormones, sleep patterns, getting familiar with our new day-to-day routine, mood variations such as irritability or guilt - but sometimes they don't. These things fluctuate, or they tend to get worse before they get better. We often struggle for months, even years, with the adjustment of adding another human to the family. No one teaches us this shit - we aren't given handbooks to help prepare us for what is about to come (well I guess there's this book). *Here, read this - you guys will all master motherhood now.* We are basically left to figure it out on our own, and we do in the end, it just doesn't mean that it's easy.

For me, the first couple of weeks were by far the most difficult, mainly for the physical rawness of child birthing symptoms. When I was able to lose the granny diaper, when my bleeding stopped, raw nipples came through to the other side, and when my Oxycontin prescription (sadly) came to an end; that is when I felt more able to deal with everything else. My mind and hormones were still all over the map, but at least my vagina was healed enough for me to (somewhat) deal with them.

The first couple of weeks is a true test of your overall mental health and your ability to cope with the life that presents to you. During this time, you really land your bearings and engage in, perhaps, the biggest shift of your entire life. It is new, it is foreign, and it scares the shit out of you. You are in the thick of it right now.

The hope is that as the days pass, our mood swings will not be as sharp and our fogginess will eventually begin to lift. Hopefully, you will have gotten to know your new little stranger a bit more during these initial days, and will perhaps have begun to see changes in them too.

During these first couple of weeks, aside from all of the breastfeeding/bottle feeding shenanigans we previously talked about, you are in survival mode. Your baby basically eats, shits and sleeps for most of the day. They do tend to sleep away the majority of the day, something crazy like sixteen to eighteen hours per day. If it's possible, try and nap when your baby naps. Ya know…

if the immense anxiety, itchy hemorrhoids and perineal pain allow. These days, these moments. Keep moving forward. Keep feeding despite the pain, keep soothing baby despite the never-ending cries. Keep soaking up the support within the community that *is* around you. You are amazing and your efforts will never go unnoticed.

You are almost over the two-week hump. Only 86 more days to go.

Tip: Tape a positive affirmation that you have written about yourself to the fridge. Make a dedicated commitment to read that aloud to yourself when you get up every morning. Stand there and read it over and over until it shifts something within you. It may not always, depending on the day, and that's okay. You will have tough days. Try adding words like "I am trying to believe that..." or, "I am having a hard time with this affirmation right now, but...".

Listen to your body, it will tell you what it needs. Not enough? Be accepting of the help from others or go get a therapist (seriously). There is no shame in checking in with someone who can monitor how you are doing.

You are fucking human and it's okay to be transparent.

One of the biggest challenges I faced during pregnancy/postpartum was:

_____

_____

_____

_____

_____

_____

I feel fucked up about:

_____

_____

_____

_____

_____

_____

_____

_____

My Wednesday night circus show looked a little like this:

_____

_____

_____

_____

_____

_____

_____

My anxiety can fuck off any time now. If I could talk to my anxiety I would say:

_____

_____

_____

_____

_____

_____

_____

If you feel like you are a fucking mess and you need some time and space to vent, you can do it here:

_____

_____

_____

_____

_____

_____

_____

_____

_____

_____

_____

_____

_____

What helped me through this time was:

_____

_____

_____

_____

Something compassionate I could say to my new mom bod would be:

_____

_____

_____

_____

Advice I would give a girlfriend going through postpartum struggles would be:

_____

_____

_____

_____

Fuck Societal Pressure.

Breastfeeding? Great. Not breastfeeding? Also, great. Co-sleeping? Sipping wine? Soothers? Flu shots? Play dates? Pets? Daycare? One thing you will notice during this whole journey is the continuous criticism that you will receive from society. Literally, from everybody. You will quickly learn that you cannot do anything right. If you choose to breastfeed then you are babying your little one, if you are bottle feeding them then you are a bad mom denying them of natural nutrients. Do you like wine? You're an alcoholic putting yourself before your child. Don't drink? You're an uptight loser who has no fun or social life. If you co-sleep with your baby then you are endangering your child, whereas, if you put them in their room alone you are neglecting them. Store bought diapers versus cloth diapers. The list goes on.

But, if you read this and acknowledge that we, as women, are here to lift each other up along this challenging journey as opposed to judging and degrading one another, then you are already on the right track. We are here to relate, as opposed to disagree, with one another. We will feel the pressure from society. We will soon learn that it is extremely difficult to make decisions about what is best for us and our child, and we will learn even faster that ridicule quickly follows any decision.

It is at times like these that us women need to stick together and be understanding with one another's choices. From a mother to a mother, a female to a female, we must seek to support one another's choices and decisions, despite whether they differ from our own. We have enough judgement from the rest of society, we do not need it from our fellow motherhood community. Natural shit, expensive organic shit, over the counter knock-off shit… whatever, dude. If the four-thousand-dollar bottle of lotion or the cardboard-like all-natural diapers make you feel better because some celebrity put their face on it, then buy it. Do whatever you need to do to make yourself feel content. The next mom should do the same. Buying no-name reusable milk stained shit on the community buy and sell page to save a buck because kids are fucking expensive? Good, me too. Focus on your own shit and respect another woman's right to do the same.

The *best* is when we are judged for the name that we picked out when naming our child - the one that we loved and chose specifically for them. *Why is the name that I have given my child any of your concern? It shouldn't be. Why? Because it's not your fucking kid.* Receiving flack from anyone? Then a nice, smiley "fuck you" will do just the trick. Carry on with your life and with your beautifully named offspring. Judgemental fucks.

Think this is bad? This is the judgement and pressure that comes along with having a *baby*; someone that can barely even keep their fucking eyes open. *Think about when they actually start to walk and talk and grow and gain interests.* The judgement that comes along with that shit. Screen time, parenting styles, eating patterns, blah blah blah. iPad? Unparenting mother. No iPad? What type of hippy seventies sick shit is this? If you spank your kid, you're an abuser. If you don't, they are a menace with no discipline. Picky eaters, public tantrums, haircuts, hair dye, hair styles, clothing choices, fucking Halloween costumes... OMG... it's ridiculous. And if you are one of those moms who posts shit on Facebook or social media mom's groups, then prepare for backlash before you even hit the 'send' button.

May you all have the power to let your middle finger be louder than the fucking mommy controversial debate club.

Society has the power to bring us down. These are people and pressures, often behind screens, that have the ability to judge and bring us to a lower level than we ever knew we were capable of falling to.

We feel pressured to have it all together, especially the size of our asses soon after we deliver our tiny human. The societal obligation to be a certain dress size is unfair to us, as females, and is super fucked up in nature. We are surrounded with images of picture-perfect bodies, regardless of where we are at in our childbearing journey. Our hips widen for a reason, our boobs grow because they serve a purpose, our skin is literally tearing apart because our body is expanding at an unexplainable rate. These things have a *purpose. What's your fucking excuse, Doug?*

Every single bodily change that we undergo throughout pregnancy and childbirth happens because it serves a functional purpose. These are the natural symptoms associated with the phenomenon of housing and growing human beings, yet we feel pressured to diet and hit the gym as soon as we are able.

Fuck anyone out there who makes you feel not good enough for how you look after you just birthed a baby. It could even be months or years after you have delivered your baby. Maybe you don't even have a fucking baby, I don't know. Bodies change, they are supposed to. We are already too hard on ourselves during this overwhelming transformation, we do not need it from anybody else. We may not be completely approving of our new mom bods, and we don't have to be. We don't have to like everything that we see, but we can start by acknowledging the immense work that we just underwent to make another human life possible. Fuck the ignorant prick who is too dumb to acknowledge the same. *My dog collar is going off the charts right now.*

We also feel pressured to get up and shower every day, looking presentable to only the cat who greets and enjoys our presence. We feel the need to promptly arrange beautifully taken family/newborn photos ten days after our body was literally cut in half. *Don't forget to post these perfectly airbrushed photos on Instagram and Facebook, just to make all the other new disheveled moms feel like shit.* Thanks for that. For me, there was not enough makeup in the world to even attempt newborn photos. *Pictures? A selfie? What are you, high?*

We feel that we should be well enough to do multiple loads of laundry, clean the toilets, and have a hot meal waiting for our hubby when he returns home from the hardest and most exhausting job on the entire planet. His job, ya know, is the hardest and most exhausting job on the entire planet. Sorry, not sure if you heard me: *It is the most intense and exhausting job that has ever existed on the entire planet.* He'll tell you himself, day after day, even as you sit there in your sad milk-stained bathrobe with rat nested hair and bags under your eyes that droop to your cheekbones. He'll *still* tell you. And I know what you all are thinking: *Oh, hi. I'm sorry, did your penis just deliver a small mammal while being ripped to your chota only to be stapled back up again by a smokin' hot nurse?* I hope you shit yourself, too.

Motherhood should be easy, folks. Besides, all we do is sit around in our sweats all day and play with a baby. (If you haven't figured me out by now, I am being *extremely* fucking sarcastic.) And I can truly tell you that during this postpartum period, sitting around in those sweatpants, petting your cat with only a load of laundry to do and a toilet to clean, is perhaps one of the most difficult jobs of all time. (I am totally not a cat person, but I thought petting your 'lamb' would be a bit too weird.)

Do yourself a favour and surround yourself with people who are positive and who are able to lift you up. Positivity is a state of mind. Forget the perfect cake you are supposed to bake for your husband's birthday, or if you feel the need to acknowledge the other children in the household. Store bought crap is just as good. Seek those people who admire the good in you and support you in your decisions. It will be life-changing.

Society can be a real bitch sometimes.

Tip: Buy the sweatpants a size bigger. It may help you feel better. Take a break from social media. Can't do that, ya Instagram addict? Then post a picture of a ripped Playboy bunny modeling naked somewhere outdoors in a snowbank with the caption 'loving my new postpartum bod,' just for shits. The humour may take the edge off.

Values about raising kids that are true to me are:

_____

_____

_____

_____

_____

_____

Societal expectations that make me want to rip my
fucking hair out are:

_____

_____

_____

_____

_____

_____

_____

People and things and pressures who piss me off:

_____

_____

_____

_____

_____

_____

_____

Real things that I wish I could say that are not socially appropriate are (Tell us how you really feel):

_____

_____

_____

_____

_____

_____

_____

_____

Shit I secretly recite in my head when my husband has the fucking man flu:

_____

_____

_____

_____

_____

_____

_____

_____

_____

_____

_____

_____

_____

_____

The Countdown.

You are about two weeks postpartum. Every week that lies ahead will be similar in its routine, but ever so different in detail. You have survived the first couple of weeks, all which contained the firsts of many 'firsts'. You have possibly met with nurses and lactation consultants, you have avoided your self-inviting in-laws, gotten through the toughest learning curve - breastfeeding, and have hopefully ridden the hormonal wave somewhere closer to calmer waters. Be proud of yourself. This may not feel like a milestone in itself, but to know you have mastered all of those things without more than a three-hour stretch of sleep appears pretty badass to me.

Your baby will still continue to sleep the majority of her days, and we will surprisingly adapt to the lack of sleep that we receive as a twenty-four-hour milk service. We will notice our baby becoming slightly more alert during this second week postpartum, having their little eyes open for slightly longer periods of time. We will hopefully feel more connected with them at this point, as our mother-child bond continues to strengthen over time. Be patient here, it takes time to get to know and befriend a stranger.

We hope that after a couple of weeks we are slowly starting to get into somewhat of a groove. We're becoming more familiar with nursing and feeding schedules, as well as nap time and sleep patterns. Not that a two-week-old baby has a *predictable* nap time, but hopefully we will learn what to expect as far as duration of their sleep and what we can do with ourselves during these times.

We should see a decrease in our overall physical symptoms such as vaginal distress, breast soreness, and bodily swelling. With every day that passes, we hope to feel slightly better on the physical end of things, like a literal train wreck recovering from its damages. At this point in time, our blood clots will have come to a halt, but granny pads may still be our staple. Our nipples will still be tender, but the bleeding should have subsided by now. If you had a c-section, don't expect to be fully healed. You were cut in half, remember? That incision will feel like a fire on fire for many days ahead. Even if we think we feel we have healed from the surgery, don't forget about the multiple layers of skin that were cut into below the surface of the only scar that's visible. These incisions take time to heal. Be gentle on yourself and abide by the doctor's guidelines on this one.

We are pretty hypersensitive during this time. Here we may notice initial bum rashes, jaundice, baby acne, and every other sign that leads us to think that our baby is not well. We are in a very protective mama bear mode during this stage. We tend to be overreactive to most things, as we should be. Our baby is so fragile at this age and all we want is for them to be perfectly healthy and okay. These things can take a significant toll on our emotional health, for we worry about them and often fear the worst if we suspect something isn't right.

Keep those resources and health line numbers handy. You are forever welcome to seek feedback and advice for yourself and your little ones.

I hope you are enjoying some baby snuggles and the comfort that comes with couching for hours at a time. Even though we are tired and without shower, nothing feels better than a sweet little babe resting on our chests. Not there yet? All good. Still struggling to find cuddle time between feeds and cries? It's all good. These things are not written in stone with time restricted obligations. They take time. Be true to yourself. This shit is hard.

Like really hard.

Pressure Points.

Around this two-week mark is when women often start putting pressure on themselves about their bodies. (Already? Yeah, I know. 'Member that fucked up society thing?) We think that we should be dropping *all* of the pounds by now, only having delivered a baby a couple of weeks ago. Thanks, society, for the fucked-up standard that we feel we need to live up to. Such a pitiful shame. As if we do not have enough stress going on in our current day, we feel (for some effed-up reason) that we will only be accepted with a tinier waistline. *You just birthed a baby hippo – be kind to yourself.* It's easier said than done.

But, on the flip side, honey, if you do know a famous bodily fourteen-day cure, let a sister know. I will help you patent that shit and we can get rich together.

I would be a hypocrite to remind you to stay patient, for I am an overweight, stretched out feline, as well. It is hard to show self-compassion at any given time, let alone this being one of the most vulnerable times in our lives. I get it. But I am also trying to lean into a more forgiving place in my life, one where I strive to not be so hard on myself. It's been a journey and a constant battle for sure, but I believe that the power of working toward that self-forgiveness will pay off. If you should practice self-compassion at any point in your life, practice it here.

Not sure what self-compassion means? Look it up, google it, attend a support group for it. I don't care. But do something, it will be life-changing. The expectation of fitting into your pre-pregnancy jeans this soon after childbirth just because the baby is physically on the outside of you, is simply unrealistic. Don't be so hard on yourself. I know it's difficult, but that time will come. Be patient with yourself.

And for now, enjoy the time where you can lounge in your sweats and still rock the oversized white cotton panties from the hospital. Who gives a shit if you've even brushed your hair or teeth today? Your plants don't care, nor does your goldfish, and Netflix sure as shit can't smell you through the television. So, kick back, Sparky, and enjoy not having any obligation to leave your house for a while. Forget the outside world, driving, traffic chaos, registrar line-ups and overpriced grocery trips. You are right where you need to be.

I always thought there was something disturbingly special about this dark and 'ugly' stage. We can safely hide out in the comfort of our living room without having to get up and get ready every day to mingle within a society of people that we don't even like. There is something to be said about just being *us* without any obligation to the outside world. It is where we can sit on our floor in confidence, with unbrushed teeth and uncombed hair, boobs out, coffee in hand (or wine, who the fuck is even there to judge and know the difference?), while watching recordings of MTV soap operas. We still feel those societal pressures, of course, but when we are able to disconnect and focus solely on our sweet little miracle, it's like time stands still and society no longer exists. Cherish those moments. They pass way too quickly.

The sun will rise and then it will set. We get up every morning and do it all over again. We power through the nursing, which at this point I must add, may take up to sixty fucking minutes at a time. We change the diapers, we attempt to make dinner, we find ourselves binge watching scandalous chick flicks on the tube. We have a couple of cries throughout the day, we may return a text or two, and we wait for what seems like forever for our partners to return home from work (that most important job on earth may keep them a little while longer for overtime). We do the sleepless night-time routine thing, feeding endlessly around the clock, constantly wondering what the fuck we have gotten ourselves into?

And, when the morning arrives, we will do it all again.

Why? Because we just do. Because we need to, because we want to. But mostly, because we just do.

Take Your Time.

If we have been hibernating inside our home for what seems like a while now, we may attempt a walk outdoors with our wee one, though we may not. If we do, it may only be to the mailbox at the corner, or maybe we're that mom of four kids who has already taken our two-week-old to Mexico. Whichever it is, it's still an outing and it still provokes particular emotions within us. First time outing? It's scary. We are hesitant to venture too far from the security of our living room, the place where our ass has made a permanent imprint on the chesterfield, and where our breast pump patiently awaits our return. If you are a new mom who got up the courage to venture outside within the first couple of weeks, I applaud you.

Those are foreign waters that take some *balls*: not man flu kinda balls, but more like *warrior badass mother fucking female reproducing kinda balls*. Good for you. The mailbox is a big accomplishment. You slowly waddled all the way over there only to realize that you forgot the keys, 'cause, well, baby brain. Then you waddled all the way back just to turn around and do it again. Good for you. Reward yourself with a fourth cup of coffee or small glass of wine. It's only 8:00 a.m.? Good thing time doesn't count on mat leave.

You may even be up for visitors at this point, or a random coffee with the nosy neighbour that you have been blowing off for the last fourteen days. You will likely plan these between feeds, to avoid having to whip your oversized breast out in front of a random. You will learn quickly that those feeds now determine your life. So, get used to that. You will know when you feel up and ready for company or meet-ups. Trust your hormones on this one. If you feel like socializing, then reach out. If you do not, Dr. Phil is a one-sided gig. Whatever. You do you. You know yourself best.

Take your time. These things are not meant to be rushed. Even though you might be regaining some of your mobility and temptation to venture from the main floor, know that these first days and weeks are still very wearing. Take your time and listen to your body. It will tell you what it's needing.

Sun up, sun down. The weeks are rolling now. Pretty soon, your little bug will be one month old. Holy shit, how the hell did that happen? I'll tell you how that happened: sleep deprivation and a whole lotta hormone fog. That's how that happened. But as the hormones settle and the fog continues to lift, hopefully we will be able to be a little more present in the coming days. It truly is amazing to watch a small human grow and develop in their newest days.

At this point, around the one-month mark, your baby will start to turn their head from side to side. It is *incredible* watching their little motor skills develop. They will also start cooing and making unique sounds and may even begin to recognize your voice. Let's hope to the fuckin' Lord they sleep longer stretches during the night, too.

It's funny how we get over-the-top excited about head turns and cooing noises, better yet the lack of yellow puss streaming from our incision. Boy, how times have changed. Who would ever have thought that a new discounted Costco vacuum or a fuzzy footed onesie with a zipper would give us the same amount of excitement as a previously scored eight ball and a forty of vodka? Shit, are we old. We're fucking parents now.

Our roles have shifted significantly. Our world is no longer about us. We have other little people to put before us. This is hard. It's like a tiny little piece of our independence has been stripped from us, shredded into little micro pieces, lit on fire and spread into the winded air. It's gone. We can no longer jump in the car and take off to the mall, hit the pub on Wednesday for wing night as we please, or take our sweet ass time pruning in the bathtub. Those times are over.

This was a huge shift for me, personally. I used to be someone who would jump on airplanes when I felt like I missed the beach. I would travel with friends, explore countries alone, and would do everything on *my* schedule. I felt trapped not being able to do that anymore. My oldest is five, and the satisfaction is not the same escaping to Walmart when we feel the need to run away from it all. Mexico vs. Walmart. That's a sad, sad, exchange. We grieve that part of us. She's still there, not lost forever, just put aside for a bit. Our priorities are different and the selfish parts of us become frustrated and resentful of that. We may even resent our little ones at times for this. As if it's their fault that we had premarital sex while drunk at a fucking football game. Their smiling faces and cute little button noses make it all so much easier, but that doesn't mean that we do not miss our old selves extremely.

Bonus? We will probably benefit from the Walmart Mastercard.

What About Sex?

The one-month milestone is a big one, not just for that sweet little baby of yours, but for you as well. This is the time, ladies, between now and that sweet, sweet six-week mark, that we will be given the all clear and the go-ahead to resume sexual intercourse. Yup. S-E-X. You know, the initial drunken adventure that shredded your vagina all the way up into your anus in the first place. Ya, that one. Wanna do it again?

That is either going to be a big turn on for you, or it's going to be a big *no fucking thanks*. Whether you are ready to be intimate with your partner or you have them sleeping in the spare room with an invite only room rule, the choice is yours as to when you want to revisit that part of your relationship. I personally avoided my husband for months. I never wanted him anywhere near my vagina ever again. *You son of a bitch. Like, love you, but take you and your business to the shower.*

Be true to yourself here, ladies. Just because your vagina is *physically* able to manage an erect external object, does not mean that you are emotionally ready to do so, and that is perfectly okay. (May I then suggest the "womanizer"; a handy little vibration tool that may do just the trick?) But don't let this deter you either. Maybe you are like that crazy-ass Ruth over there, got all the whips and chains and dildos perfectly set up and aligned, ready for her and partner to get back in the saddle - super horned-up and ready to fire. All the power to you, Ruth. I can't wait to buy your book.

I will tell you, though, that a penis is like some fucking jacked up out of hibernation anaconda on a scavenger hunt for a crippled, vulnerable, injured little rabbit. Your vagina is the rabbit. It will hunt you down and it will get you. I'm telling you, that thing's got teeth. Deadbolt your bedroom. Wear a helmet. I dunno. Hoard some bear spray. That mother fucker is coming for you.

My point here: Your post-delivery vagina = your rules. Do whatever you want. No sex, vanilla sex, holding hands, sexting, abstinence, weird swing domination shit... I don't care. Listen to your gut (vagina) on this one, and do whatever feels right. This is your call. Nobody else's.

One month has quickly and dreadfully passed. Roughly 72 days to go.

It's a Tiny Person!

As we stumble through the next few weeks, month one and two of our wee ones' lives are quite different. You will see an increase in their motor skills, as they continue to hold and grasp small items. They will soon be able to hold their heads up, wiggle about, and may even start to roll over. Their smiles will become bigger, as will their diaper loads. They are starting to develop their little personalities quickly, gaining some essential smarts, too. So much that they could most probably pick your nipples out of a line up.

These little gaffers will be stuck to you like glue - you are really just a big security blankie who stores endless amounts of milk, accessible at any given time, regardless of the hour or situation. Put in a nice way: *we are their fucking slaves*. We will do whatever they want whenever they want it. We are brainwashed, basically, into thinking that we must run around catering to these little aliens who simply just lay there and exist. They are absolutely exhausting for the amount of time that they spend sleeping the day away. Yet, we are personal assistants to them and will pretty much bow down to any one of their demands. We should actually get uniforms, recite a routine speech and sing a song when the sun rises and our mornings start. That would be classic.

Despite them being constantly attached to us, we have the pleasure of watching them grow and experience life through the eyes of a truly innocent being. We get to bear witness to every new beginning that they have. Even as their slave, we are a beautiful witness to the constant changes happening before us.

They are only weeks old and, still, they consume us. They are babies who shit in their own pants and smile about it. That, right there, is consuming. These creatures haven't even started walking yet - or better yet, drug dealing in grade school, stealing our minivan or knocking up the neighbour chick. Oh my God. Think about the wine intake I'll need at that point. If I struggle to survive cute little *coo*s and *caw*s at this point, then sweet Jesus, somebody better take the fuckin' wheel.

What's Up, Doc?

You will see your doctor or OBGYN at your six-week check-up. This might still be an overwhelming and emotional time. It has only been six weeks. That little bean is still fairly new. If you have any questions about your recovery or concerns about the baby, this is a good time to ask them.

If you had a c-section, you will probably be cleared for driving - if you were like me, you will probably have been driving the whole time anyways, because who hires transportation services to take your other children to and from school when your partner is busy at work? *Not this fucking mom.*

During these weeks, we hope to see some weight gain on our little ones, bigger appetites and hopefully longer sleep patterns. Your baby is probably beginning to master somewhat of a latch, making it easier for her to eat more efficiently. We hope to become more comfortable in our ability to soothe our crying babies, nurse them in public and feel confident enough that we look like we have our shit together in the eyes of others.

We might not have our shit together in the eyes of others, most chances are that we do not... Hence the Fuck Societal Pressure chapter in this book.

Lunch Time.

I avoided breastfeeding in public with both of my children. It was terrifying. I would time outings around feeds and escape to the isolating back corner bathroom stall when dinner time struck. I was worried about judgement, ridicule and the embarrassment of someone seeing my hideous beast of a nipple. It was a very anxious place to be, having to hide the beautiful and natural act of feeding my baby whilst, at the same time, the slutty eighteen-year-old gets old man stares and attention from having her tits and ass cheeks hung out of her crop top. My exposed boob that is currently keeping a human alive is unacceptable, all while hers is not. Fuckin' twisted, man.

I see other women whip their boob out at restaurant tables, picnic park benches, even on the public transit bus, and I think: *good for you. I truly wish I would have had that willpower.* It's hard to live with no regrets. I wish I would have been able to be stronger in some of those moments, truer to what I believe in, and more dismissive of other people's judgements. But it's hard in those moments when you feel so vulnerable. Public feeding = bathroom stall. For me, it was about survival.

Pat yourselves on the back, you have somehow survived to the eight-week mark. Two months in and over halfway to our 100-day mark. I hope this slippery slope has been getting easier for you. I truly hope you have been able to witness some significant shifts within yourself, and, well, frankly the last thing I need is a bunch of people suing me for false advertisement of this book. Let's hope we've all made small gains.

Every gain we make, no matter how small, is still a gain. Washing your hair on day number nine, better yet your ass, is still a fucking gain. Personal hygiene, washing clothes, doing chores... those are all gains. Those take energy, they take strength. Even on the days when that is all we have accomplished, we have still accomplished something. Do not underestimate the power of folded socks, or the fact that we just took the chicken out of the freezer and set it on the counter to make it look like we actually had dinner figured out for the night. Those are all big things! Raw chicken removed from the freezer, and folding a bedspread, are big things.

Get into the Groove.

Weeks nine, ten and eleven - these weeks tend to blend together. This is the time when your babe is between the two and three-month mark. Still a blur, as you are going through the motions, but hopefully you are starting to feel more comfortable within your own groove. You may have your own little morning routine, and an evening bath ritual as well. Routines can be important, as they help us to feel structured and more in control. No routine or rituals? All good. You are figuring it out just as well as the rest of us.

During this time, your baby will continue to reach for foreign objects and will start to follow you across the room with their eyes. They will start to giggle and may even start to suck on their thumbs and fingers. They are starting to put on some weight and may appear chubbier in their arms and legs. Their cooing and cawing will become louder, as will their sweet little cries.

Know that at any time it is perfectly, one hundred percent okay for you to place your baby in their crib, close the door and walk away if they are crying at a level that literally makes you want to climb a mountain just to jump off the top of it. Adult timeouts are a thing, ya know. Utilize them. Take a moment, inhale deeply, exhale the same, and recoup yourself. This is normal. You are safe. You will get through this.

Go grab your baby and carry on.

You've got this. And if you think you don't, then there's wine for that, too. I've heard vibrators are good stress relievers, as well.

Sleep Training.

Women often wonder when is an appropriate time to sleep train (getting your baby sleeping through the night in their own bedroom). You may have heard of the cry-out method. This is a controversial topic dependent upon beliefs, cultural ideas and our own laziness to strictly implement a consistent night-time routine. Some women feel anxious to have it done *now*, even though their babe is only a number of weeks old, while others argue that sleep training should not be done before at least six months of age, or at all, seeing as how we are animals by nature and find it appropriate to sleep with our young.

Personally, I am a pretty big fan of co-sleeping. Both of our boys slept with us in our bed for about the first eight to ten months, basically until they were able to sleep through the night by themselves. I am a sucker for co-sleeping and loved the comforting aspect of it. It was annoying at times for sure, as it would hinder the quality of my sleep, but just like everything, I knew that it wouldn't last forever. I actually started to dread the day they would be too big to not want to cuddle with me. And that day comes very quick.

There is no right or wrong way to look at this issue. Many women choose to play it day-by-day or week-by-week, as things can change ever so quickly. Do your research if you want; many people prefer to understand the logistics of sleep training. You may want to weigh the pros and cons of crib sleeping versus co-sleeping, trying to determine how emotionally dependent or anxiously attached their child will be from either method. You will find a ton of research on the topic, for and against each decision. There is a slight chance you will even feel worse and more overwhelmed after looking into this. You're damned if you co-sleep; you're fucked if you don't.

As with most of the advice I have been giving you women throughout this book - *you do you, mama.* Sleep training, co-sleeping, bassinet, crib, fucking blow-up mattress, fucking water bed. I don't care. You know why? Cause it's not my fucking kid. Is your kid alive? Yeah. Do you want them in your bed or not? Maybe? Ok. Can you function on little sleep? Are you okay with your baby self-soothing back to sleep? Are you trying to do the best that you know how to do? Great. Good. Perfect. That is all that we need. That is your business and nobody fucking else's.

If your baby is still eating every three to four hours during the night and you find yourself pissed off at the mom who told your their two month old sleeps for ten hours straight, just take a deep breath and another shot of wine, because chances are she's fucking lying or... chances are she's basically just fucking lying. Neither one of my sons slept for more than four to five-hour stints until they were about ten months old. Maybe that is not always the case, but it is definitely not abnormal either. With every week that passes, we hope our baby sleeps a little bit deeper and a little bit longer. Hopefully, we are able to sleep between their nightly feeds and feel half-some normal when the morning strikes. Coffee will be endless here. Baileys optional. Sweats mandatory. And hopefully there's fucking bacon served.

Hang in there, ladies. You are *so* close to the 100-day mark.

Grow Baby Grow.

A milestone that I remember around this three-month mark is the baby's first time in the swimming pool! Usually, people wait until around the two to three-month mark to expose their child to the ever so disgusting communal bathing centre. Some sooner, some later. Most babies love the water, so it could definitely be a highlighted event in the household.

I recall the look on my husband's face when I rolled out in my new post-baby bathing suit. He thought it looked like an oversized polka dot diaper, but was being polite, of course. He always compliments me, and I love him for that, but I also could have fucking slapped him. In hindsight, it was most likely my own insecurity wanting to cover up my overly stretched mid area. *"Do you know how much money I paid for this trendy high-waisted bikini? They are so in right now."* The look on his face when he saw the *actual* price of the high waisted 'diaper' was priceless. *And that was on your credit card honey, not my secret one.*

Did I mention that every woman should have a secret credit card? Helpless trooper.

As your baby continues to chat, wiggle, squirm, and maybe even break dance, you too will hopefully be gaining some more personal momentum. Not all the time of course, but you might be able to get through a load of laundry or a minor poop session without crying endlessly, like in previous months. This is a huge breakthrough, ladies. We can actually get through a task without having a chaotic breakdown!

This is big.

This is change.

This is progress!

Who the Hell *am* I Anymore?

We may notice changes in ourselves as hormones continue to shift and settle. For example, hair loss (due to falling estrogen levels), or changes with our skin and nails. We may also feel well enough to resume physical exercise. Our moods will still fluctuate. We may feel pretty stable for hours at a time, and then completely low and depressed for others. This is something that was more prevalent before, but persists as we go through our days. Just because our overall hormonal output has somewhat leveled in force, does not mean that we will not experience up and down wave-like spells that hit us like flying pheasants blindfolded in the night. It's like Halloween in the middle of July. Or better yet, some frickin' Blair Witch Project on a random fucking Tuesday. These swings can be scary, and at times, unexpected. Is it any coincidence that most moms are witches on Halloween? We should make a female version of Freddy Krueger. Just sayin'.

The emotional imbalances that fluctuate throughout these weeks are a whirlwind of uncertainty. They will have you questioning yourself and your ability to manage life as a mother. You are doing every little bit of normal. And you're doing it just fine. You got this.

As your babe gets older and continues to grow, the three-month milestone appears to be a big one. It is as if they are transforming from an infant baby to a bigger baby. A more mature baby, bigger than the infant one. A timeline milestone, if any.

We are somewhat used to having a dependant by now. We are familiar with sleepless nights and constantly feeling like shit. A good indicator of actually feeling better overall, though, is that the baby is growing bigger, is eating more productively and is actually sleeping more soundly throughout the night. Aside from our physical healing, we need these components to progress in order for ourselves to feel somewhat better.

Over the last few months, we have spent the majority of our days alone. The baby doesn't really count here. We have not been to work at our once regular schedules, our partner is typically away for most of the day and our friends have their own lives with their own adult shit to live and deal with. As lonely and isolating as postpartum and maternity leave can be, we have spent a large amount of time alone, with ourselves. We have experienced happy thoughts, as well as those thoughts that are unwanted. We have had to sit and cope through emotional distress. We have felt all of the feels and have tested our patience in more ways than anticipated. It's been a mix of ups and downs, triumphs and defeats. It has been savouring that hot cup of coffee with the 5:00 a.m. news, or pounding back shots of red wine to cope with the screeching sounds of endless cries.

It's called coping.

We have probably had a lot of time to think and reflect, not just on our struggles and current life situation, but on ourselves and who we are at this point. We have been there to watch our little one grow and develop, have changed way too many diapers and have been there to wipe their tears. We have rocked them, soothed them, cuddled them, and played with them. We have celebrated milestones and have adopted a new baby talk foreign language that is *super* fucking annoying to others. We've been there through all of it. Us. Alone. As moms. We've shown up. We have felt proud, excited and so overly grateful. We felt those things. We were present for those things. We may feel like we've been stuck in our sweatpants within the walls of our living room for the past three months with nothing to do and no one to really talk to, but, oh mama, how we've grown.

They say that uncomfortable situations are where change happens. Nothing about pregnancy, delivery and raising dependent humans is one hundred percent comfortable.

I wonder what you have, or are, learning about yourself during this time. You have spent more time alone with yourself here, in a very vulnerable state. More than, perhaps, ever. You, too have grown. You have shifted perspectives, adopted new roles, and developed new strengths. You have evolved.

Have you had the opportunity to reflect on these times? What have you learned about yourself?

The hope in approaching our three-month postpartum mark is that we will start to re-see pieces of ourselves that were possibly lost along this journey. Not lost, per se, just hidden under the foggy hormonal bliss that blurred the lens of ourselves and the world. Even if the flabby tummy still exists and the stretch marks are an everyday reminder of our beautiful and challenging journey, maybe there has been something deeper within us that has shifted. Maybe we have started to see our bodies differently, maybe we have adopted a new form of gratitude. Maybe we can start to view things from a more compassionate lens as we approach the other side of the 100-day postpartum mark.

Maybe this is a time when we are able to sit and take a deep breath and watch our baby sleeping soundly in their bassinet (or blow-up fucking waterbed). We lean over quietly in the dark, watching their peaceful little porcelain face resting so sweetly, and can see their little chest breathing up and down ever so lightly. They are so quiet. Peaceful. We feel love. We feel attached. We feel bonded.

And then… we suddenly queef. Just kidding.

…we feel attached. We feel bonded. We realize that it is moments like these that have us feeling overwhelmed with gratitude. We love them - their soft skin, their little hands, their perfect little ears and their innocent horrendous cries. This is what it is all about. Motherhood. We listen as they breathe in and out of their perfect little round noses, we feel their warmth. We momentarily forget about whatever it is that we have been through.

They are our children and we are their mothers. This is it. That's all we have to know for now.

The sun will rise, and then it will set. We will do it all over again tomorrow because we are their mothers.

You survived.

Congratulations. You have made it to the 100-day mark.

Tip: Take lots of pictures! Or buy a journal where you can record baby's "firsts" as well as your own personal journey. Photo books make great keepsakes. There are many treasurable times here that you will want to remember!

Engage yourself in mom and tot play groups, solely for the purpose of adult interaction and getting out of the house. Also, remember to choose your infants' friends by their mothers who match your wine drinking habits. Also, buy the expensive over-sized polka dotted swimming 'diaper' in every single fucking colour available.

Things I have noticed about myself during this time are:

_____

_____

_____

_____

_____

_____

_____

If I had sex at that six-week mark I would describe it as:

_____

_____

_____

_____

_____

_____

_____

My vagina would describe it as:

_____

_____

_____

_____

_____

_____

Some of my biggest learnings have been:

_____

_____

_____

_____

_____

_____

My favourite go-to wine during this time has been:

_____

_____

_____

Looking back on the last 100 days, some highlights for me have been:

_____

_____

_____

_____

_____

_____

_____

_____

_____

Some memorable moments have been:

_____

_____

_____

_____

_____

_____

_____

_____

_____is the approximate amount of daytime
hours I have spent on Netflix.

My favourite Dr. Phil quote would be:

_____

_____

_____

_____

_____

_____

Things I still want to say to my nipples are:

_____

_____

_____

_____

The limit on my secret credit card is:

_____

You Survived.

Now what the fuck do I do? Well, nothing special there, Sparky. You carry on, mama, as you would. You have done an amazing job thus far. You keep rocking the badass job that you have done until now. You know the one - feeding your baby, taking adult timeouts when needed, having sex as you want, day drinking with Dr. Phil, and not giving a fuck what other people think. That would be the recommended starter pack.

The 100-day mark does not mean the end of an era. It may mean the end of this book, but that does not mean the end of an era. The 100-day milestone marks a segue into the many months ahead. It signifies that perhaps the hardest days are behind you, mostly the newest and scariest ones, also the rawest and most disgusting. These were the initial days that you birthed and met your baby, developed a relationship with them and somehow got it together enough to keep them alive. I am hoping, as you reflect on the past few months, that you are able to acknowledge the challenging times, as well as the joyful ones - those filled with milestones, love, and gratitude.

There will surely be challenging days ahead, but challenging in different ways. We will shed many more tears, have many more meltdowns, have many days of feeling low and alone and many times where we feel completely overwhelmed and out of control. But now we get to do it in the absence of an oversized granny diaper and without cracked nipples. I hope you have mastered a few ways of managing those. Call a friend, ask for help, take deep breaths and keep that chin up.

We will experience days where we are head over heels in love with our children. We will laugh and play, teaching them new things by exploring the world around us as we build so many memories. It's an up and down roller coaster kind of gig. It's a fucking ride that nobody could ever have prepared us for.

Motherhood is the most rewarding, yet the most challenging, job that we will ever do.

You ladies have delivered strangers and have been committed to getting to know them. You have provided a home for them, security, and the food supply that has literally kept them alive since birth. You have groomed them, protected them and loved them, all while putting those needs in front of your own. Even on the darkest of days, you have still done all of those things. That is the definition of motherhood. That is the definition of love.

My hope is that this short read did not deter you from having children, rather it allowed you to view yourself as much stronger than you ever knew yourself to be. My hope is that you recognize that you are not alone in your tears, anxieties, isolation, and oversized granny panties. We are all in this together, and we will survive it together, too.

My hope for all of you is that you will continue to put one foot in front of the other, wiping away one tear at a time and powering through every day that lies ahead. You should be proud of yourself for all that you have done and everything that you have survived.

On those doubtful days when you feel lost, alone, and have no idea what to do or where to go, remember that there is someone else in the room. And that someone else thinks that you're *perfect*.

Carry on as you have been. You are a queen bee, a rock star, a mother effin' Goddess. And maybe even a prophet, to boot.

And for the Lord's sake, keep on top of your recycled wine bottles, they add up pretty quick.

Tip: Day drink like you've never day drank before. You'll be back to work soon, and that will be a very, very sad day.

Personal reflection about how I actually fucking survived this:

_____

_____

_____

_____

_____

_____

_____

If I could leave a message in a bottle for a pregnant lady to one day stumble upon, it would read:

_____

_____

_____

_____

_____

_____

_____

The sun will rise and then it will set, and The First 100 DAYS will happen somewhere in between.

Closing.

I started writing this book about five and a half years ago when I was on maternity leave with my first son. It was more of a journal, really, my outlet to release thoughts onto paper when I simply didn't know what else to do with them. My struggles at the time were mainly around the physical aftermath of birth, bodily issues, and some mood fluctuations that left me feeling alone. As time passed and things became easier, I felt less of the need to write, and more of the need to connect externally. So, I stopped writing. There was no need to anymore.

It wasn't until I became pregnant with my second living child, about five years later, where I revisited my journaling. My husband and I had four miscarriages between our two boys.

My second son is our little miracle babe. I did everything in my own personal power to get him here today. I did weekly acupuncture, massage therapy, physiotherapy, dietary changes, stress leaves, all to find out that his, too, was a naturally high-risk pregnancy.

I had developed a bizarre dual lobed placenta that put both me and the baby at risk. I spent the first and third trimester on a modified bed rest, being overseen by a high-risk outreach team from my local hospital during the latter half. While my own individual nurse, equipped with weekly home visits and bi-weekly ultrasounds was nice, the anxiety of losing a baby at any given moment,

183

was not. The anxiety during this time was perhaps worse than any anxiety I had felt at any given point post birth (at least the baby was already out).

It wasn't until that pregnancy with my second son that my thinking started to shift around the aftermath of childbirth. Originally, I associated bearing a child with stretch marks, a broken vagina, and a couple of unexpected tears. It took four losses, a high-risk pregnancy and two trimesters on bedrest to realize that pregnancy is much more than physical. I was alone, crying on my couch in my sweatpants - yes with my donair and an extra side of hummus - but I was alone. I felt disconnected from reality in an unexplainable way.

The trauma that I experienced from previous loss was weird, because unlike other traumas that we experience in our lives, this was a trauma that I experienced within my own body. It was profound. And it was then that I realized the importance of community. I saw people see me. I felt involved in related groups. For once, I experienced a connection within my isolation; it saved me.

It was after my second born that I revisited this journaling thing, but this time with a different twist on things. I wasn't twenty-seven and accidentally knocked up anymore - even though the aftermath of that pregnancy was nothing but the truth. I was now in my thirties and entrenched in the emotional turmoil that accompanies this experience. I wasn't 'cute' and pregnant anymore. I was anxious, irritable, and scared. (And overweight. You gain a lot more with your second.)

I have been pregnant six times and have birthed two living babies. I have had one vaginal delivery and one scheduled cesarean. I don't have pets, even though I refer to myself as a lamb sometimes. Actually, not true. My son had a fish once that he named Sarah Pluto. Don't ask. I'm just a small-town girl from Alberta, Canada, who went to university to become a helping professional. I am not an author in any sense of the word, but I am a mom. One who has real experiences and real emotions, and a ton of shit to say around this whole birthing and motherhood phenomenon.

When I went for a D&C one random morning, they asked me what I wanted to do with the baby's remains. I feel choked as I write this, for even though it was years ago, it feels like it was just yesterday. I couldn't comprehend that question at the time. But I can now. And after what I have been through and what I know now, my answer to that question may have looked a little bit different.

I remember every single thing about that day: what I wore, my husband's hourly work schedule, even the grocer's name on the plastic bag as I threw up in the truck on the way there (it was Safeway, by the way). What I remember most, besides the interactions with the most comforting staff and absolutely every single particular detail inside of the operating room, was the community that came with that. It was on that day, with

185

my first baby now gone, that I became a part of *that* community. I was involved now. No one understands how big that community actually is until you are actually in it. I appreciated the support, so connected with groups that were involved with pregnancy loss. I felt comforted and supported being surrounded by like-minded people, ones who generated relatable vibes on an uplifting level. It was a safe place to share a somewhat mutual understanding.

The understanding and acceptance of these groups and individuals is what carried me through each and every loss. Community is powerful.

I decided to write this book because no one talks about this shit. Had I read something similar to this on the days when I was feeling low, maybe I would have felt comfort in knowing that other people feel this way too. Maybe I would have given myself permission to not compare the dark, emotional way I was feeling to the perfect Pinterest mom who has it all together on Instagram.

We all *know* that pregnancy and the postpartum period is challenging, but we don't often speak about it. Maybe we do. Maybe it's just not loud enough.

I wrote this book because I wanted to be transparent with myself. I didn't want to sit around and act like everything was cookie cutter A-Okay. Because it wasn't. And why do we always have to lie and hide behind the truth pretending that it is? It's like posting a flawless picture of ourselves on social media and acting like there weren't twenty-four imperfect ones before that. Who are we kidding? And why? And who knows, maybe you had an amazing experience with the whole childbearing process. Maybe you didn't get one ounce of anxiety the entire time, maybe you opted out of the epidural and smiled throughout your whole vaginal delivery. If you did, I am truly and honestly amazed and so utterly happy for you. But mostly amazed. Because that takes some balls. Who are you, like, Satan's warrior chick? Or maybe just a robot? I envy you.

But if you didn't, that's totally okay too. That's why I'm writing this, because us women need to be more honest with ourselves and with the people around us. And, maybe when we are, we can actually create some sort of change. Maybe we can connect with others, we can seek help, we can see the value in what's actually happening.

Not acknowledging the truth does not change our reality.

This shit is hard. It's the hardest thing you may ever actually ever do in your entire life, but trust me, it won't kill you. You may think it will, but it won't. Bootcamp hungover, now that shit has a more probable chance of killing you. Don't be doin' that shit. Tempting fate, right there. It's not worth it. But yeah, childbirth. Yeah, it's fucking hard. You are strong, though. And you will get through it.

So, as you read this in your fat pants, know that you are not alone. Know that you are an amazing human being. Know that you are worthy, that you have a voice. That you have a right to set boundaries and for them to be respected. Know that your thoughts, feelings and emotions are valid. Know that you have been through a lot, regardless of the journey. Know that you matter. And know that you are needed by that little bundle in a beautiful shitty diaper. You created them. You are needed and you are loved.

We are women and we need to stick together and support one another during this time. So, if you see a woman in need, help her. Connect with her. Relate with her. It's that simple.

I wish for everyone reading this nothing but health and happiness, as well as the strength that is needed to overcome whatever daily obstacles are thrown your way.

I hope…

…that you learn and grow as a human being, recognizing your own strength and resilience.

…that you will support other women as opposed to placing unnecessary judgement.

…that you learn to appreciate your body and everything that it undergoes to create life.

…that you can find self-love and learn to practice self-compassion.

…that you dismiss pressure from society about the mother you think you 'should' be.

…that you continue to strive for the beautiful life that you were given.

…that you learn to love the shit out of your children.

If you have struggled with infertility, and/or pregnancy and infant loss, I hope you are given the strength to overcome those challenges.

This book is meant to highlight the beauty of childbirth and the strength of women, while also speaking to the rawness of it all. So, know that when I speak the truth, even with harsh and disturbing words and imagery, there is still beauty within that realness. It is within our own bodies that we have created life. It's real. It's hard. It's disgusting. It's beautiful. And it's time we started talking about it.

I love my children more than anything in this world, and I would do all of this sick shit over again in a heartbeat.

I feel proud of myself because:

_____

_____

_____

_____

_____

_____

If I had an 'aha moment' along this journey it would be:

_____

_____

_____

_____

_____

_____

_____

_____

My hopes for myself are:

_____

_____

_____

_____

_____

_____

I feel grateful for:

_____

_____

_____

_____

_____

_____

_____

My hopes for other moms would be:

_____

_____

_____

_____

_____

_____

My own million-dollar piece of advice would be:

_____

_____

_____

_____

_____

_____

_____

When I doubt myself I will be reminded that:

_____

_____

_____

_____

_____

_____

_____

Wishes I have for my baby are:

_____

_____

_____

_____

_____

_____

Go back to the *Mood Stuff* chapter and read aloud the very last journal statement to yourself.

Words from my Fellow Mamas..

"It's like the time my tits let down in the middle of a K-mart shopping trip. Some of those things you just never forget. I haven't delivered a baby in over 29 years, but there are still specific things that come to mind when I think back to those days. Weight gain: gross. Having sex again: don't even think about it. I recall feeling fearful when I became pregnant with my second baby, as I had pretty bad postpartum depression with my first. It was all very overwhelming and pressuresome - the "image" that women must portray throughout this journey. It was defeating at times."

- Anonymous

"I try not to look through a negative lens when I think back to the days of postpartum, but honestly, there were not very many pleasant experiences. I recall feeling super stressed and overwhelmed. I didn't have that immediate bond with my baby when I held them for the first time, and I felt pressured to, because that's what we are "supposed" to feel as women holding their babies. But, how could I? The baby was swollen and covered in juices, and I was so exhausted from hours of labour, not to mention the epidural and all of the other pain meds. That's how I met my baby for the first time. 'Hi, I haven't slept, I don't know you, and I'm on drugs'.

I got in the vehicle when leaving the hospital and thought: 'now what?' I had no idea what I was doing. I was not only embarrassed from shitting the blow-up tub during my water birth, now I was overwhelmed and scared, too. I slowly learned that you just grow to figure it out, but it takes a while to get to that place."

- J.M.

"I have two kids, and even though the second came three short years after the first, I forgot EVERYTHING I did for the first. When do I start a nap schedule? What food do I feed them first? So, FYI - that happens. My experiences were very different, both painful and beautiful at the same time. The first time I pushed a 9.5-pound baby out of my vagina and her shoulders got stuck. After that, I opted for an elective c-section. I recommend the latter.

Things I've learned on this crazy journey they call motherhood: (i) try to coordinate maternity leave with a friend, it can be very isolating; (ii) don't make too many plans for the period after birth... I spent the first 8 weeks topless in my living room breastfeeding; (iii) lots of people get the 'blues' after childbirth, I hear it is awful. I got mad... so in case that's you, I think it is normal, and it will pass; (iv) for the vaginal births - freeze wet maxi pads to ice your vagina after; (v) you may need to advocate for yourself, if you want a c-section, push for it. If you need more drugs after the c-section, push for them!; (vi) my boobs can shoot breast milk up to two feet away when a baby cries."

- L. L.

"My baby is three weeks old. She is a pretty awesome bubba and I am extremely grateful for her. That being said, there is

absolutely no way to prepare yourself for the level of pain that brought her here.

It started on a Tuesday morning, contractions about every ten minutes apart. It wasn't until the following morning that I got to the hospital. The nurse working at the time was nasty and asked me if I've tried other pain management options like a warm shower, breathing, and exercise. I was like, what the fuck? Exercise?! Like, I didn't sleep for 24 hours and then she tells me the pain from the contractions is not even bad because they are only ten minutes apart. I received a shot of Gravol and morphine and was sent home. Later that evening, the contractions got more painful and I started to labour in the bath. I called my husband. I had to immediately go on my hands and knees buck naked and just rock back and forth as my husband watched over me. I started crying saying, "I don't want to do this anymore." The level of pain was indescribable.

Needless to say, I made it to the hospital and got the epidural. Best decision ever."

- S.P.

"After four consecutive miscarriages, I vowed I would never complain about motherhood when I was finally blessed with a baby. But as a new mom I quickly learned that such complaints were actually more pleas of help and triumphs as resiliency.

I was inadequately prepared for the resentment I felt towards my husband. As a new father his lifestyle and wellbeing appeared to be seemingly unaffected. I, however, was recovering from an emergency c-section, struggling with nursing woes, was socially isolated and enduring unthinkable fatigue. I hated him for it.

This motherhood shit is hard. I am forever thankful for the experience but have learned there is room for us to share our struggles and our gratitude all at once."

- A.S.

"I'm currently in the trenches. As I write this, my second kid has just turned four months old. Part of me wants to offer advice to expectant parents but the other part of me says to not offer any because, honestly, you just can't prepare for this. We all arrogantly think we can, but we just can't. It's not possible. It's not quite the same as packing for your first trip to Europe and you're like, 'Oh yeah I have an idea of how this is going to go. I've never been but I've seen it on TV.' No. You literally have no idea.

Growing, birthing, and raising a tiny version of you and your partner is the most extreme sport you will ever participate in. Period. I'm sure you're going to tell me that you know what I'm talking about because you're the reigning pacific octopus mud wrestling champion, but you only do that shit a couple times a year. Eff that, I'm wrestling mine every day and I never even trained for it. Because you can't."

- T.G.

"Getting pregnant was not a romantic experience. I ended up convincing my husband to have sex for 14 days straight just so I didn't miss 'the window'. Once successful, it was a long ten months of weight gain, being unable to sleep, unbearable heartburn, wearing a panty liner 24/7, throwing up, being out

of breath walking up stairs, and having trouble bending over to put on my shoes.

When my son was born, I was overjoyed and so excited. I tend not to remember the sleepless nights, crying while my baby cried because I did not know what to do, having to pump all the time to keep my supply up, having an emergency surgery to get my appendix out, and not having much of a social life for the first nine months - and let's add wanting to divorce my husband on a weekly basis.

I quickly forgot all about those things and when my son was 11 months old, I got pregnant again. Not sure why I would put my body, mental state and relationship through that again, but I'm days away from having my second and am very excited for baby number two to be born."

- R.M.

"I dreamed of becoming a mom. I knew there would be challenges, but no one prepared me for this. 24 hours of labour, pushing, a c-section and my son is here! I longed for the moment I'd have my son on my chest, but all I could do was vomit from the pain. Okay, that didn't go how I expected! What's next? We need to clip his tongue. Okay. He won't suck, won't latch and won't take a bottle. Off to the ICU. Okay. Now my son isn't even in the same hospital as me. OKAY.

A few hours later, I join him and sit by his side with tubes and wires coming out of him. I cry. I've got blood and bodily fluids all over me. I am not allowed to shower, I smell and have a melted mushy padsicle. I have no shirt on, and the nurse is helping me manually get 1ml of colostrum out of my breast which took about an hour! So, this is motherhood! It's dirty, smelly, embarrassing, exposing, hard work, sacrificing, and overwhelming with a mix of every emotion in the book. And the fucked-up part is that I would do it all over again for my son. He is my world and I am so lucky to be his mom."

- G.W.

"I felt really challenged when I had my second baby. Having the first one is hard. Your life changes, but then boom, you have your second baby and it suddenly got 283 759 291 037 449 times more difficult.

I remember walking up the stairs in the first few weeks after having our second daughter. I stopped halfway up, looked at my husband who was sitting on the couch and said, 'What have we done? We had it so good.' Quite literally overnight I had a baby who needed to eat every two hours and a two and a half year old toddler who needed attention every 0.3 seconds. We struggled at first. Just a few weeks before, I had 'me' time, a lovely bedtime routine, and time to watch Netflix. Now we were each taking turns bouncing on an exercise ball holding a newborn 'till our backs felt like they might break. It was rough. Fast forward a few months and we were in what they call the four-month sleep regression. It felt more like an apocalypse. We were zombies.

Was it all bad? Not really. I mean we loved our little babies through every twist and turn. It's a rollercoaster, though - just when I found my groove was usually when everything changed anyway (new milestones, sleep regressions, etc.)."

"I remember feeling panic and anxiety wondering if I could be a mom, if I was good enough to take care of another human. The day my son was born I swear something just came over me and I took control. Two days post-delivery with my first, I put a mirror on the floor, I stood over it and had a look to see the damage. I needed to desperately understand how the hell another human came out of my body. I was humbled and surprised that, other than a lot of swelling, I was okay.

With both of my sons' pregnancies I felt calm and in control. As I enter week 31 with this pregnancy, a daughter (what the heck do I do with a girl? I don't even know how to change a girl's diaper!), I feel so many emotions. I cry during commercials and when I look at my sons, and I feel more and more in love with my husband than ever, while at the same time feeling so distant because this pregnancy is physically tolling on my body and I have nothing left for him at the end of the day. I've felt secluded more often than not from friends.

This motherhood thing is amazing, and sucks at the same time. I miss my boobs, I miss sleeping in, I miss days without somebody else touching me. I can't imagine what my life would look like without my boys and soon-to-be daughter. I feel overwhelmed some days, but I show up and give these kids every ounce of love I have, and also everything I never had, to prove I can do it."

"The first few months are all about survival. For you, your baby, and your marriage. Nobody said it was easy, but some

days are really hard. Your entire life changes, your marriage changes... but not all for the bad. You literally learn how little sleep you need to function, how much coffee you rely on, and how much wine is safe to drink while nursing. You find new friends with new common interests. You figure out how to vacuum, fold clothes and make dinner, all while having a baby attached to your boob. It's tiring and it's messy but if you ask me, or any mom, we wouldn't change it for the world. Maybe it's all the wine we drink now that's making us forget those early days."

- K.C.

"Kids were a segment in my life that I was not prepared for. The new norm: I rush to my husband's office to pick him up, drive 45 minutes through traffic to the suburbs where we can actually afford a nice house, rush to day-care at a cost of $3000 per month, put kids in their coats and boots, strap them into their car seats, rush home, pray I have something ready to cook, have a kid refuse to eat and be a straight up snack bitch, clean up the kitchen, try and happily play for 30 minutes together, throw them in the bath, brush hair and teeth, throw in laundry, set out their clothes and school gear for the morning, set out my own clothes for the morning, get ready for bed, fight with kids about falling asleep in their own bed. Finally, at 9:00 p.m. I get into my bed, my husband rolls over and touches my vagina, and I feel like I could cut off his hand cause I don't want to be touched by anyone or anything, but then I don't want to be a shitty wife and not have sex with my husband. So, I take a deep breath and suck it up and do whatever it takes to

make him finish the absolute fastest. I go to sleep, get woken up several times throughout the night for pees and cuddles and waters, and maybe even more laundry if an accident happens.

Friday rolls around. My husband and I pour extra-large drinks, maybe even take an edible, and crawl in bed fantasizing about what we would be doing right now without kids. We both know we would be rich and well-rested, that's for sure.

You will be a goddamn slave to your entire family for the rest of your life. That's the truth."

- Anonymous.

"There are four little babies I think of often when I reflect on my pregnancy, childbirth and the 'fourth trimester' (postpartum). My daughter, S. (2011), my angel, A. (born and passed in 2012 at 20 weeks of pregnancy), my second daughter, K. (2014) and my littlest, Z (2016). Of course, the stillbirth holds a special place in my broken heart, but it was the birth that makes me reflect on my postpartum so differently, and in some ways more deeply. I have been a jumbled confusing mess of extreme joy and postpartum depression all while evolving into the badass single mom I am today. There are days I question my competence as a mother. I have asked questions like: will I ever stop bleeding? Is the c-section scar infected? Will I ever fucking sleep? Am I messing up this sweet kid? Is her REAL and BETTER mom going to walk in and take over?

I am so glad that I bonded with my cute baby girls enough to love, feed and nurture them, even throughout these scary thoughts. The questions have since changed in nature

205

(although I still wonder about bodily functions a lot) but caring for and loving my three little girls so damn much has somehow kept me going at a successful pace.

The rawness of new motherhood has of course faded, but has it ever taught me to embrace the mess of it all in a way I am so grateful for. The 'mess' no longer includes maxi pads, breast pads and bed pads for me. But I look forward to the next stage of motherhood where I will be coaching my own daughters through their stages of needing all the different friggin' pads."

- R.W.

About the Author.

I grew up hating to read. Not sure if I've ever finished a book front to back in my entire life.

Instead I liked to write. I liked to be creative and artistic. I drew. I painted. I dreamed.

I started traveling the world at a young age and very quickly developed a passion for the world and all of its diversity, cultural aspects, ethnicities. No matter where I went, no matter how long the duration, I always ended up back at home. My safe place.

I got married and we had two boys. It was hard, challenges I was never prepared for. Bearing children is raw and disgusting and real and overwhelming and emotionally taxing on our whole being. What I have realized is that no matter what country or land we hail from, no matter our wealth, race, or status, we as women are all the same. We bare children. It is hard and disgusting and emotionally taxing, and it is our safe place.

I am the proud mother of two little boys, I am a professional in my community, and I have a passion for wine and travel. I chose to write a book because I thought there were too many real and darkened moments that are commonly shared but are never mentioned. I wanted a place to express myself, with the hopes that others could read and relate.

I believe in transparency and the ability to "own our shit". We are women. We bear children. It's a disgustingly beautiful thing.

I may have written the book, but I still hate to read.

If you are wanting to connect further, please visit www.thefirst100days.ca